# Praise for
# *Differences in Common*

. . . . . . . . . . . . . . . . . . . . . . . . . . . . . . . . . . . . . . . . .

"A grand gift to families no matter what their child's age or abilities. Marilyn Trainer's essays are superb—rich with all the joy, humor, sadness, hope, pain, and love that make up family life. This book is a valuable contribution. Everyone should read it!"

> Martha Moraghan Jablow, *author of*
> Cara: Growing with a Retarded Child

"This rich collection of essays displays a rare ability to share intimacy, to convey tenderness, misgivings, or simple pride. In tracing the growth of a little boy into manhood, these pieces also offer a look at the changes in society at large. Gutsy, plainspoken, and filled with a rejuvenating sense of humor, the gems in *Differences in Common* make for wonderful reading."

> Margaret Lewis, *Editor*, Down Syndrome News

"*Differences in Common* made me smile, made me feel sad, and made me feel a oneness with all parents of special children. I highly recommend this meaningful collection in which Marilyn Trainer gives us keen insight into her indomitable spirit, and the true value of each human being."

> Claire D. Canning, *parent, and author of* The Gift of Martha

"An excellent book for parents and everyone with a desire to understand the triumphs and challenges of raising a child with a disability. Marilyn Trainer has the strength and ability to reach out to other parents and professionals who do not share her convictions and to understand their concerns, too."

> Joyce Glenner, *Association for Retarded Citizens*
> *Montgomery County, Maryland*

# Differences In Common

## Straight Talk on Mental Retardation, Down Syndrome, and Life

Marilyn Trainer
Foreword by Helen Featherstone

WOODBINE HOUSE • 1991

362.19
T

For information regarding bulk sales of this book, please contact:
Woodbine House
5615 Fishers Lane
Rockville, MD 20852
800/843–7323

Cover photography: Charlie Brown

Some of the essays in this collection have appeared elsewhere, in slightly different form: "I Wish I Had Given a Better Smile," "Two Hours without Ben," "He'll Never Sing at the Met" (under the title "Raising a Retarded Child"), "It's Not Funny, But. . . ." (under the title "Down's Syndrome: Parents Can Still Smile, Sometimes Laugh"), and "Is the World Ready for the Graduates?" in the Journal Newspapers; "Those TV Commercials Are Passing Up a Natural" and "Ben on Ben" (under the title "Insight from a Retarded Child") in the *Washington Star*; "Phantoms" (under the title "Reflections: Whatever Happened to Mickey?"), "A Joyous, Painful Graduation" and "He's Lucky, This Little Boy" in the *Washington Post*; "The 'Sunshine' Kid" and "Nursery School" (under the title "Ben and Normal Nursery School") in *Sharing Our Caring*; and "Finding the Holiday Spirit" (under the title "Finding the Christmas Spirit") in the *Sentinel*.

**Library of Congress Cataloging-in-Publication Data**

Trainer, Marilyn.
    Differences in common : straight talk on mental retardation, Down syndrome, and life / by Marilyn Trainer ; foreword by Helen Featherstone.
        p.  cm.
    ISBN 0–933149–40–9 : $14.95
    1. Down's syndrome.    I. Title.
RJ506.D68T73    1991
362.19685842—dc20                                                    90–50503
                                                                      CIP

Manufactured in the United States of America

1 2 3 4 5 6 7 8 9 0

# Dedication

......................

This book is dedicated with much love to Allen for his expertise with the photocopier, the malfunctioning typewriter, the faulty ribbons, etc., but mostly for his infinite patience day in day out, and to Ben and his friends, who have a remarkable way of bringing out the best in all of us.

# Contents

· · · · · · · · · · · · · · · · · ·

# Foreword

## *Helen Featherstone*

........................

L ast night, after reading *Differences in Common*, I dreamed about
Jody, my own severely handicapped son, who died ten years
ago. It is a shock to write "ten years ago"; it doesn't seem that long. But
each year, when Jody's birthday approaches and I think how old he
would be, my imagination stalls. How can I imagine a nineteen-year-
old Jody? It is as impossible as imagining my other children middle-
aged, or myself at seventy-five.

In my dream our daughters had taught Jody to walk and to talk.
"What did he say?" my husband, Jay, asked when I told him of the dream
in the morning. Still half asleep—and half immersed in the dream—I
tried to remember. The question seemed so obvious, and so important:
often I had wanted desperately to know what Jody thought. We who
are word-driven people, who hang on words written and spoken, how
intently we wondered what words Jody might have spoken if his tongue
and vocal chords had cooperated. Yet in my dream his particular words
were unremarkable. "Ordinary things," I told Jay. I could only actually
remember one word: "Yes," articulated clearly, spoken with the as-
surance of a born speaker. I didn't even know what question had
elicited this ringing affirmative.

My report disappointed me a little: I wanted to have dreamed "real"
words for Jody, words that might tell us a bit about what he had thought
all those wordless years. (I wrote 'inarticulate' and crossed it out. Jody's
smiles and sounds communicated delight, surprise, amusement,
warmth, pain, and fellow feeling very clearly. I'm not sure he was
"inarticulate.") But as I thought more about that clear unhesitating
"yes," I felt satisfied. Coupled with Jody's ambient smile, the dream
message seemed to shout hurray.

i

In the dream, the talking came first and seemed almost natural. It is the moment of walking that I remember best: Liza, Caitlin, and Miranda, partly hidden in the doorway, whispering and giggling to their brother, launch him toward me, and he totters uncertainly into the room, taking at least ten steps before folding into my arms. I had no idea *how* the girls had taught Jody these things, but I was thrilled not only by the upright Jody but by the children's conspiracy, and I was delighted that Liza and Caitlin had included Miranda, who was not actually born until after Jody died.

I see this dream as a kind of meditation on Marilyn Trainer's book. *Differences in Common* evokes clearly the experience of living with a child with disabilities. When Trainer describes her agonizing resolve not to burden her own mother and father with the knowledge that their baby grandson had Down syndrome—or "mongolism," in the grotesque parlance of this bygone era—she shows us how our children's disabilities and our response to those disabilities shape relationships with the child's grandparents as well as the lives of brothers, sisters, parents, and, of course, that of the disabled child himself—how they make a difference for the whole web of family.

A serious disability limits communication in obvious and not so obvious ways. Ordinary parenthood brings many women closer to their own mothers by putting them deeply in touch with an experience that is in some ways the same for both generations; but mothering a child with a disability immerses us in worries that most other people have not faced and this sets us apart. Our parents, as Trainer reminds us, are of a different generation, raised with different—and often more tragic—attitudes toward disability. Even more important, they are *our* parents, and often they feel for us the same protectiveness we feel for our children. My mother, because she longed to spare me the heartbreak and fatigue she was certain Jody's care would bring, wanted us to place him in some sort of residential care. She did not pressure me, but she did mention her hope several times. It wasn't something that we could talk comfortably about together; I knew her impulse was rooted in love, but I felt sick at the thought. I knew, when I let myself think about it, that Jody's disabilities gnawed at her heart in ways, and

ii

to a degree, that she did not show me. That realization pained me so deeply that I did not probe it.

Perhaps because Trainer has written these essays over the long run of her son's life, she is able to evoke specific moments and longings that she felt in Ben's early years and to carry others who have walked in her shoes back in time. In "Inklings," she describes the uncertainty she felt, early on, about whether Ben would ever learn to *think*. She finds her answer when Ben, just two, toddles into the kitchen and sees her sweeping the kitchen floor. After sizing up the situation he goes to the kitchen closet, finds a dustpan, and kneels down to hold it for his mother. Trainer is ecstatic: Ben has observed, remembered, anticipated, and he has put it all together. He has thought! "A burden was lifted from me that day. . . . His seemingly simple action seemed to me a promise of good things to come." Most parents of children with mental disabilities have such moments, moments in which their children seem to cross some important divide and demonstrate to their families that, disabled though they surely are, they are more like the rest of us than they are different.

I have not been the parent of a teenager or adult with handicaps: Jody died when he was nine and a half. But because Trainer speaks believably about the childhood years I do know, I follow her trustingly into the realm of adulthood, sharing with her in emotional 3-D, for example, the sickening terrors of her son's two-hour disappearance on his way home from his job. I remember the terrible night I spent trying to locate my eighteen-year-old daughter who had disappeared somewhere between Detroit's Metro Airport and our home near Boston. (At 4:00 a.m., a trans-Atlantic phone call informed me that she had dozed off on the plane, slept through the Boston stop, and woken up over the Irish coast, an hour short of Gatwick Airport.) So like all parents, I know a bit about what these dark hours are like. But I know, too, the limits of my knowledge. Because Jody was Jody, and because he died young, there are subtleties of Trainer's two hours that I have not tasted:

> We worry about our normal children to be sure. But the added vulnerability of our youngsters with mental retardation also adds to our agony when something goes

iii

wrong, because it is our choice to let them go, and in so doing, we know we are choosing risk.

The most vivid character in this book is Trainer's son Bennett, a young man with Down syndrome who is funny, exuberant, creative, occasionally pathetic, and always very much alive. Our libraries, bookstores, and movie theaters give us very few such characters, very few chances to get to know an *adult* with mental retardation.

The omission is significant, both for families and for social policy. Children with mental retardation grow up to be adults with mental retardation. Given the relative duration of childhood and adulthood, there are probably more adults than children with mental retardation. But how much do most citizens worry about these adults? How often do they think about the fact that schools, which once provided them with education, a daily round of activities, and a place to meet friends, disappeared from their lives years ago and that some never connect with jobs or services that fill the void?

When our baby is born with a handicap we are buffeted by our feelings of terror, despair, guilt, and inadequacy. As the years pass we have to move outside ourselves to find services and schooling for our child. For a growing number of us in recent years, the basic services have been there: when we have struggled it has been for something extra. (Of course this isn't true for everyone, but for many it is—in 1991 mothers do not so often hear, as I did in 1975 when I inquired about schooling for Jody, "He sounds like he should be home with his mother.")

But if schools now make some provision for our retarded children, it is a lot less clear, especially in times of economic recession, that the wider world does the same when they reach adulthood. Reading Marilyn Trainer's account of her search for a job for Ben in the months following his high school graduation, we realize how empty the promises of education and vocational training can be in the absence of real jobs. (This is of course also true for non-disabled students facing joblessness in our increasingly callous society, but it hits the disabled with extra force.) Education for what? The Trainers faced the awful possibility that Ben, after sixteen years of schooling and four successful job placements, might have to sit home and vegetate for years, even decades. Eventually Ben's mother found him a job—indeed, a job that was conveniently located and well suited to his skills and interests. But what if she had been less assertive, less sure that Ben *could* hold his own if given a chance? What if she had given up after ten rejections? What if she had had a full-time job herself?

Young (and not so young) adults like Ben Trainer need decent jobs and leisure activities with friends as much as my son, Jody, needed an early intervention program and a teacher who discovered how much he could benefit from music therapy. In some ways, although comparisons are odious, they need them more, because adulthood is a life sentence.

The last nineteen years have visited serious permanent disabilities on both my son and my mother. I know that my experience is not typical, and it may be that I am simply oblivious, but my travels with Jody rarely brought me face to face with rudeness or hostility. Although I had to try to rise above what Marilyn Trainer aptly terms "the cringe factor"—the relative strangers who assured me that I was "so wonderful" or that I was doing "such a marvelous job"—it seemed to me that most of the attention Jody attracted was kind and well-intentioned. And whatever uncertainty or discomfort our friends, neighbors, and relatives may have felt in private, they supported us constantly and in a thousand ways. We survived the wrenching loss of Jody's death because of the support and love we got from each other, from parents, children, siblings, in-laws, friends, and from the people we barely knew whom Jody's life had touched. At his funeral we all knew that we needed to sing the Beatles song, "I Get By with a Little Help from My Friends."

But I cannot paint such an upbeat portrait of life with the disabilities that Parkinson's disease brought to my mother. People *did* stare as we helped her in and out of restaurants, airplanes, and public bathrooms. They sometimes looked frightened or confused. They did not as often offer the kind of casual help—a door held for a wheelchair, a friendly greeting to the disabled person—that helped to make life with Jody a series of new connections with strangers. My mother's disabilities—she made peculiar comments, had difficulty with all aspects of self-care, and saw things that other people did not see—embarrassed people in a way that Jody's did not. Adults with mental disabilities are not cute as Jody and Ben Trainer were at nine years of age.

We cannot wheedle from a reluctant society programs and jobs for adults with mental retardation by arguing that these interventions will save the taxpayers money in the long run or that with proper training these men and women will be nearly normal. Our case for such programs must rest on the importance of creating a society that cares for people—even those who aren't cute—and gives them a chance for growth, human contact, and self-respect.

We may also say that we are prudent to vote for services and work on attitudes—our own as well as those of other people—because we may ourselves, as disability groups so trenchantly remind us, be only Temporarily Able-Bodied. And even if our own minds and bodies are spared, we are almost certain to love someone who will have a serious disability at some time in his or her life.

And here, among other places, *Differences in Common* serves us well, for it helps us to really *know* Ben Trainer, an adult with mental retardation, as we could not know him if we simply met him loading groceries into our car at the grocery store. In knowing him as someone who loves his cat—dead or alive—and hates dress shoes, who has nourished friendships over more than a decade and endured the death of a beloved girlfriend, we see vividly how much he is like us and our other children and why he needs a job and opportunities to do interesting things with friends. We come to care intensely about this need, and about creating a society that will meet it.

# Introduction

. . . . . . . . . . . . . . . . . . . . . . .

In no way is this a How To book, and in no way is it written by an expert. Rather, it is a reaching out—a hoped-for connection—to those who have known the despair and the joy of loving a child who is different. It is a reaching out also to those who know little or nothing about children with disabilities, particularly children with mental retardation.

Most of the essays which make up the book are ostensibly about our son Ben, who has Down syndrome. The essays cover his life from birth into young adulthood. They also feature his friends who have Down syndrome.

Writing this book evoked a lot of old memories, some very painful, some joyous. And I began to realize that many of my dredged-up feelings were not unique to me. It's true that Down syndrome is a crucial factor in our family's life, but the themes of the book, I believe, are universal and will strike a common chord with all parents.

As you will discover, some of the essays were previously published. When I first began writing them, I had no idea whether or not editors would consider them favorably. If something hit me that I thought would be meaningful and touch somebody—awaken minds and hearts—I wrote it up and sent it off. When my essays were accepted and received with enthusiasm, I realized I had found a way to advocate for Ben and others like him.

Here I should note that, as we well know, children with Down syndrome and other handicapping conditions are born to parents from all walks of life, and these parents hold various philosophies and divergent points of view. Just because we have a common bond in our children does not mean that we are necessarily going to think alike. For example, something that really drives me up the wall is the assumption by someone that I automatically share the same outlook on life, the same belief system. It is quite possible I do *not* share them, and such automatic assumptions really offend me.

I fully expect that some readers will not agree with certain ideas expressed in this book. That's fine with me. They are valid ideas, however, which I feel strongly about and believe should be brought to light.

The book is organized so that essays written some years ago are presented early on. This would explain certain terminology which may seem outdated, but . . . like it or not . . . was the idiom of the day. The essays are in a modest semblance of chronological order. I think you will agree that the subjects of the earlier essays are as pertinent today as when they were written, and that's why they are included in this collection.

I have two hopes for this book. First, I hope that after reading it some will be able to say, I understand a little better now what it must be like for families whose children are different. And, perhaps more importantly, others will say, I know just what she means; I've been there too!

*How do you remember the days before your child with Down syndrome was born? If your child is still quite young, you may look back with bitterness or longing. If he or she is a bit older, you may feel a faint nostalgia for the freedom from worry and responsibility that once was yours. Only gradually do you begin to see that in losing that old freedom you have gained something more valuable in return. One day when Ben was around eleven, I was in a mood for looking back, and this essay was the result.*

# I Wish I Had Given a Better Smile

. . . . . . . . . . . . . . . . . . . . . . . .

It wasn't a real picnic; just a few sandwiches in the park on a bright crisp day.

But picnic or not, it was a special day—our last in California before heading across country back home to Silver Spring, Maryland.

My husband and I sat at a picnic bench watching my mother and father making a gallant effort to keep up with our three youngsters who were popping in and out among the redwood trees like squirrels gone mad with spring. Imagine! Redwoods. Walking distance from home. But that's how it was in that green and peaceful park only a few blocks from my parents' home in Oakland.

Tomorrow it would be over—our glorious trip west to see "Grandma and Grandpa"—and already an awful kind of let-down feeling had taken hold. I was glad we had the park to ourselves. I would always be able to recall the scene intact, no outsiders present; my Mom and Dad, the three scampering children, Allen and me, and the green serenity. Just us.

Only it wasn't. Somebody was entering the park, up the wooded pathway to the picnic grove. Four children and two women walking very slowly, too slowly. As they came near I saw that the children were severely retarded. I winced inwardly. Why oh why did they have to come to the park on this particular day?

They came to a stop at a nearby bench and it became apparent the two women were teachers, not the children's mothers as I had first supposed, and that they were on an outing from a school or facility.

It was hard to determine the ages of the children, but I guessed that they were about twelve or thirteen years old. There were three boys and one girl.

Suddenly one of the boys indicated by gestures that he wanted to go to the restroom, and one of the teachers led him down the path to find it while the other teacher stayed with the group.

The little girl planted herself in the middle of the path and, motionless, watched the other two disappear. She was extraordinarily thin and she stood like some strange little bird poised for flight.

Waiting . . . waiting . . . her eyes glued on the path, no words. The teacher kept reassuring her that the others would be back. The child stayed fixed in silent patience for a full ten minutes until she saw the two returning and her face lit with the joy of recognition.

Tears were in my eyes, but still why oh why did they have to come on this day?

Our own children ran flying to the table, Grandma and Grandpa huffing and puffing behind them. And we settled down for our "picnic in the park." Thank goodness our children were too young and too hungry to be aware of anything unusual. No sense to have their last day spoiled by something they couldn't understand.

But pity for those strange other children reflected in the eyes of my mother and father. And I knew Allen was thinking even as I was how lucky we were that our own three were healthy, bright, and normal.

After a little while the teachers had the children take hands, and two-by-two they left the picnic area and headed toward the trees at the far end of the park. As they passed near our table the little bird-like girl turned her head our way.

I smiled at her, a bit feebly I'm afraid, and I thought I detected a frail smile in return, but I couldn't be sure. My eyes met those of the teacher bringing up the rear of the small parade, and in her eyes, I could see compassion, for the children, and for me struggling to reach out.

I watched as they made their way slowly along the path and disappeared among the redwoods. I had never before that day laid eyes upon those children. And yet, deep within me it was as if memory rang a distant bell, as if somehow I knew them. Or would come to know them.

Why oh why had they come to the park on this particular day?

Two years later our fourth child was born and we were told that he had Down syndrome. Only they didn't call it Down syndrome then; they called it Mongolism. Ben, our cherubic baby, was a Mongoloid and we were no longer observers in the park.

Now we knew about the anguish, the fear, the guilt, and the shame.

We knew the stomach-churning anxiety of how to explain it, or not explain it, to relatives, especially to ailing grandparents. We knew the worry for our other children and what "it might do" to them. We knew what it was to have strangers and friends look but not quite look at our child and not know what to say. We knew the utter folly of projecting too far into the future and becoming terrified, but we did it anyway.

And most of all, we knew how it felt to love our baby deeply and yet wish he'd never been born.

Our child had Down syndrome and we were afflicted with another kind of syndrome. "Why us? Why us? Why us?" It is a syndrome which hits virtually every family who has had a retarded child.

But that was eleven years ago and we haven't asked that question for a long time.

Today Ben is a spunky charmer who firmly believes that a world without McDonald's would be the pits.

He is what is termed moderately retarded and he is learning to read and write and he will someday be able to hold down a job, simple perhaps, but contributing. And where once Allen and I counted ourselves so lucky to have three normal children, we extended that luck a thousand times over to include Ben. To borrow a bit from an old song—he is the sunshine of our lives.

Life with Ben is, indeed, good. But it would be an acute case of "Pollyanna-ism" and perpetual donning of rose-colored glasses to say that it is always good. There are too many times when it still hurts, and that is mostly because of other people.

Recently Ben and I were quietly waiting in a checkout line and I noticed a woman staring at him with such suspicion and hostility on her face that I wanted to slap her. I didn't, of course. I put my arm around Ben and hugged him deliberately, defiantly, and I looked her in the eye until she turned away.

Mostly, people look kindly at Ben, or they try not to be obvious when they look at him, or they look at me almost helplessly as if they don't know what to say. And always when this happens my mind goes back to that long-ago day in the park.

I see myself so clearly, the family gathered round, and I feel again how it was trying to cope with the presence of "those strange children."

Where are they now I wonder? That little bird girl—a child no longer. Is she still waiting somewhere, waiting patiently for someone to return?

I wish I had given her a better smile.

Someday Ben, too, will no longer be a child. I like to think that by the time he's grown he will garner his share of smiles just like anybody else, and that he will never be left somewhere waiting . . . waiting. . . .

If I didn't think this, my heart would surely break.

# Nursery School

. . . . . . . . . . . . . . . . . . . . . . . . . . . . . .

It was our doctor who first suggested that we try to get Ben into a nursery school with "normal" children. She thought that if he could get the maximum exposure to normal children, be a part of their activity each day, and, most important, be exposed to their developing speech, it would help his own development. This was certainly foresighted thinking for the early 1970s. After all, it would be years before Public Law 99–457 would guarantee all young children with disabilities the right to a free preschool education.

Foresighted or not, our doctor's advice struck me as being good common sense. In fact, it seemed like such a wonderful idea that I naively thought everyone else would think so too. Ben has been accepted with such warmth and genuine interest by all of our friends and neighbors that it never entered my mind that there were people who would not want Ben around. I blithely assumed that the personnel of any nursery school would find Ben as fascinating a child as we did and welcome him with open arms. It was in this innocent state of mind that I encountered for the first time the awful anguish of having my child discriminated against because he has mental retardation. It is a sobering experience.

The woman at the first school I called had a voice full of smiles as she described all the wonderful activities provided for their children. When I told her that Ben was retarded, the smiles dropped from her voice and she said they "don't take children like that."

The second school—where some years earlier I had sent my elder son—gave me the run-around about having to get special permission, checking with county officials, etc., and calling me back. The call never came.

The third school cut me off at the word "retarded."

I sat by the phone crying, waves of pain washing over me. They hadn't given Ben a chance. They didn't even know him—his bright grin, his easy comprehension, his eagerness to please. They wouldn't give him a chance.

The hurt was deep and acute, and then it changed to anger! Maybe they didn't want Ben, but somebody somewhere would want him— want the challenge of him. There had to be a place for him and I was determined to find it.

As it turned out, it wasn't only determination but a good bit of luck that opened the door for Ben. An acquaintance told me in passing conversation that she was going to be teaching at her church nursery school that fall and the director was thinking of trying to work with one retarded child, if they could find one.

"You've got him!" I cried.

And so it was that Ben began his school life in a small nursery school which happened to be held in a church, but was open to children of all persuasions, all colors and, now, even the retarded—in the person of Ben.

Actually, we started as "visitors" toward the end of the spring session. Ben was just past three, an old man by today's early-intervention standards. He was in the class with children who were chronologically four months to a year younger then he. This worked very well. Because there was a rule requiring an "extra pair of hands" to be present when a child with a special problem was enrolled, I became those hands. Ben did not need any more attention than any other child, except with things like scissors and paste. I deliberately spent more time with the other children and let the teacher handle Ben.

In the fall we had the same system, but after several months I realized, as did the staff, that Ben would not have a complete school experience until he could go off on his own without Mommy always near. Fortunately, our public school system has an intern program that allows senior high students to spend a certain number of hours each week away from school working in an area of special interest. So it was that I "retired" and Allison came and took my place as Ben's special friend.

For the first three weeks without me, Ben moped about and wouldn't cooperate with anyone. Allison, who had never worked with a retarded child before, was very discouraged. No matter what she tried to do for Ben, he rejected her. So she changed tactics; instead of seeking Ben out, she ignored him and worked more with the other children. She would sit at a table with a puzzle or game and after a while, Ben would come to see what she was doing and to "help." In a short time Ben became very attached to Allison and gave her the nickname "Sonny." I was very moved at the end of that year when Allison told me that because of her experience with Ben she was going into the field of child development so she could work with retarded children.

The second year, Ben had grown to be so independent that he went happily off to school each morning with a neighbor whose little boy was now attending the same school. I would pick them up. Allison was replaced by Vicki, and although Ben would ask now and then for "Sonny," he soon made friends with Vicki. Vicki had done volunteer work at an institution for the retarded and in comparing Ben to the institutionalized children, was amazed at his abilities.

Everyone at the school was so kind to Ben and so interested in him. Day by day he bloomed. He fit so well into the routine that casual visitors, including a doctor and a dentist, were not aware that a "special child" was among the busy group they saw.

The children, too, had good feelings about Ben. Perhaps they sensed he was somehow younger in a way, or a little different. Whatever it was, he was very popular. When he was absent they missed him and asked about him. One little girl mothered him to pieces, but he didn't seem to mind.

Ben was in the school for over two years. In that time his vocabulary increased beyond measure, his independence grew so that his favorite phrase was, and still is, "I'll do it!" And he became completely toilet trained, even at night.

We have never had any doubt that sending Ben to a normal nursery school was the right decision for us. Perhaps nothing more dramatically illustrates this than what one of the other mothers told me as the school year was drawing to a close. Her little son, Shawn, had also been at school the year before and she was very interested in Ben. She told me that one day Shawn remarked to her in the casual way that children have, "Ben talks this year the way the rest of us do."

So even a small child could see what Ben had achieved!

This observation by one of his own peers was the crowning touch to Ben's first experience in the big outside world away from home.

*When you have a kid with Down syndrome, you can get awfully tired of hearing the word special. (Your child is so special. That's why he needs special education for his special needs.) But then something happens to remind you just how special he really is. The essay below describes one such reminder Ben gave me when he was about seven years old.*

# The "Sunshine" Kid

. . . . . . . . . . . . . . . . . . . . . . . . . . . . . . . . . . . .

You have to admit there's something pretty special about a kid who keeps the sun in his dresser drawer. It's not the kind of thing most people do—even if it's only a sun made of yellow construction paper. And while he fully realizes that it's not *really* the exact sun which does its thing up in the sky, it is a *genuine substitute* sun which comes in very handy during those times when the other one has "gone away."

He *is* special, this little boy, in the truest sense of the word. And although he may achieve his goals at a slower rate than the rest of us, he also views life with a refreshing zest and determination that we can well envy . . . and an awareness of the world around him which I hope I will never again underestimate.

Take this business of the sun. Each evening as night approached and even during the day if there were cloud cover, Ben would ask over and over where the sun had gone. We explained again and again that the sun was up above the clouds or that the sun had gone to the other side of the world to shine on other children while we were sleeping.

He wasn't too impressed with our explanations, because when it came down to the nitty gritty, it was *his* sun and it belonged in *his* sky over *his* head in *his* part of the world. And that's the way it was, in Ben's eyes anyway!

Then one day the school nurse called to say that while Ben wasn't exactly sick, he wasn't himself either. The staff realized this after he took one bite of his hamburger and then wouldn't finish his lunch.

Because I did not have a car that day, I could not go to school and get him, so the nurse and I talked for a few minutes trying to figure out what the problem might be. I noticed that the sunny day had turned cloudy, and on an off chance, I mentioned this possibility to the nurse, who said she'd pass it on to his teacher.

About two hours later an exuberant Ben alighted from the school bus and came charging through the front door carrying the sun! He was singing, "It's Howdy Doody Time" at the top of his lungs even though it was cloudy and threatening to rain. I was dumbfounded, happily dumbfounded, and I began singing "Howdy Doody Time" too.

Later a conversation with his teacher shed sunlight—pardon the expression—on the whole matter. At school the class had been study-ing some very basic facts about the earth, the sky, the wind, the rain, the stars, the moon, and of course . . . the sun. And Ben had begun thinking of these things very deeply and, as children with mental retardation are wont to do, in a very literal way as they applied to him personally.

So his teacher solved the problem with what to me was a touch of genius, by cutting out a golden paper circle and giving it to him as his own personal sun to keep in his dresser drawer for whenever he needs it!

Perhaps there is some lesson in all this, but I don't know what it is. I only know that as far as Ben is concerned, he is the keeper of the sun.

And maybe that's just another reason why he is truly special.

# Night Noises

· · · · · · · · · · · · · · · · · · · · · · · · · ·

Like many parents, Allen and I always heave a great sigh of relief when we finally get our human dynamos settled for the night. I get much the same feeling of bliss which comes from taking off my favorite pair of tight shoes.

Yet as glad as I am when the children are down and quiet, I am always drawn to their rooms sometime during the evening. I go there not because they need me, for they are sound sleepers and almost always sleep through until morning. I go there because the truth is, I need them. In the darkness of a room where I can see their small forms in the soft glow of the night light, I get a feeling of peace that comes from no other experience I can think of.

I like to sit for a few minutes and listen to them. There are no sounds so delicate, so tender, or so moving as those of sleeping children: the way their breath comes and goes, punctuated now and then by a soft kind of hiccup, and the little lip-smacking noises that always sound to me like kisses, the faint moaning sighs they make that seem to come from far away, and the delightful flopping motions when they turn over and their small arms go dangling over the sides of their beds.

There's such a lovely helplessness in sleeping children. I like to think that for these moments nothing can touch them, or me. That no outside force will ever change just the way it is as I sit there in the semi-dark and listen to them sleeping.

It doesn't always work this way, though. Sometimes my eyes are filled with tears when I begin to wonder what the world will do to them, if it will even allow them to grow up, and if so, under what conditions? I can't help thinking these things. The world crowds in on us more and more these days, and I guess I'm not the only mother who aches inside when she thinks of her children in terms of the future.

But I try to push these thoughts away and take these moments for what they are; that there are small and lovely children sleeping here and that they are *my* children. I listen to them and I look at them and

I kiss them in their sleep and cover them. And sometimes I try to picture the years ahead when they may have children of their own—something that seems utterly impossible at this stage. But I try to imagine myself as a grandmother in those far years ahead with a child or two or perhaps more who will be my grandchildren, and I know instinctively that every now and then time will stop for the little old lady who'll be me, and I'll be back again in a darkened room, with my own.

I guess it's just part of an age-old ritual, rather common-place really, the mother tending her children in the night. Millions have done it before me and millions will after me, if this old world keeps spinning. Each room is softly dark, the children are sleeping with their tender night noises, and I sit there listening and watching. An old, old scene, but it's my little piece of eternity.

# Inklings

. . . . . . . . . . . . . . . . .

When Ben was an infant and I was still pretty wounded, I made a strange kind of bargain with myself. I decided that if only he could look at me some day and call me "Mommy" or "Mama," I could endure the fact that he was retarded. It was very important to me to hold the hope that he would have the ability to at least do that—identify me as his mother just the way his brother and sisters had done. And for some reason, focusing on this hope helped me to take my mind off some of my other worries.

Of course, there were a lot of other things I'd hoped Ben would do as well, but in those early weeks I was feeling awfully desolate about the future, not to mention scared and confused. I knew even then that kids with Down syndrome were able to do more than wave bye-bye and say "Mama." That is, I knew it in my *head*. But in my *heart* I was so fearful of that uncertain future. I guess, too, I was grieving for the baby who never came—that bright, beautiful baby who would do everything ahead of schedule and whose future would be one of endless, unlimited opportunities.

In retrospect, I suppose I was feeling sorry for myself. Certainly no one had painted a dreadfully bleak picture for us as has sometimes happened to other parents. No one had so much as hinted that Ben would be little more than a vegetable and we would serve our family best by sending him away.

No, this forlorn wish was something I came up with all on my own in the dark of night when I lay awake wondering what was going to happen to this changeling baby of ours, and the rest of us too.

Many parents have had similar fears. Will our baby smile? Will our baby walk? How about talking? What about learning? Will our baby be capable of *truly* learning? Will he be able to *think*—actually use his brain to *think*?

And is there any way to know all this ahead of time?

Although there are no guaranteed answers for any child, for the most part, these questions can be answered with a resounding *yes!* Still, parents wonder and worry, and no matter how many reassurances they may have from others—even doctors and experienced parents—that nagging doubt is there.

Your child grows, and he *does* learn to smile, and sit up, and wave bye-bye, and say "Mommy," and a whole lot more. You begin to feel better; you can see for yourself that he is doing things, reaching milestones, "progressing nicely," as the experts might say.

Yet, you find yourself waiting for something—you don't even know what—something that will enable you to set your doubts aside once and for all, find a reality you know you can more than cope with.

One morning when Ben was barely past two, he toddled into the kitchen and found me sweeping the floor. He observed me for a moment and I saw him glance around the room. Then he toddled over to the kitchen closet, opened the door, reached in to pull out the dust pan, and brought it to me. Next he bent down and held it near the broom. I was dumbfounded, and then oh, how I wanted to pick him up, dust pan, broom, and all, and go dancing around the kitchen! (I guess this would be called a "Broom Dance.") That's what I *wanted* to do, but I didn't. Instead, I carefully swept debris into the dust pan as he held it for me. I knew it was very important to let him follow through on his actions. We could dance later!

I doubt that parents who have only normal children would have greeted Ben's efforts with anything more than an "Oh, isn't that cute!" But parents of children with mental retardation have a different perspective. This was a true epiphany for me.

What Ben had done was not just something "cute" in passing. What Ben had done was to *observe*—to *remember*—to *anticipate*—to *put it all together*—and then act upon it. This was *thinking*. On that particular day, it finally jelled for me. Beyond any doubt my little boy could *think!*

Now, Ben had certainly given evidence of thought before. I could hardly discount the night I went into his room to check on him and found that he had unscrewed his bottle top—those little fingers were

more dexterous than I knew—and poured milk all over his head, not
to mention his pajamas and bedding. (I guess I should have believed
him when he said "No!" to his bottle.) And the way he pouted at
strangers, but would blow kisses to those he knew and loved, showed
his ability to discriminate. Or when he realized that sliding down the
stairs on his bottom was a whole lot faster than walking down one step
at a time. Not to forget either his discovery that if you caught the cat
by her tail, she had a harder time getting away, but that she might also
turn and bite you!

Oh, Ben had a lot of things figured out, but there was something
different about his bringing me the dust pan. Perhaps it was because his
actions didn't really pertain *just* to him, or because it was a series of
actions—remembered, perceived, and anticipated—that he had to
match up, or because he showed for the first time that he was a little
kid who could see a chance to help his mother and knew how to go
about doing it. In any event, what he did was pretty sophisticated for
a two-year-old, if you think about it.

When we were through sweeping, I carried the dust pan to the trash
container and let Ben help me empty it and then I handed it to him.
He went immediately to the closet and put the pan inside, up against
the wall where I always kept it. He gave me a look and said, "Broom!"
I realized he was waiting for me to bring the broom, so I took it to him
and let him help me stash it in the closet, too. He grinned at me with
the satisfaction of someone who has done a really good job.

A burden was lifted from me that day. I was not so unrealistic as to
believe Ben would grow up to be a nuclear physicist or a Rhodes
Scholar, or enter a profession that requires exceptional brain power. I
wasn't even thinking in terms of average. That wasn't the issue; it never
had been. The important fact here was that Ben could *think*. At two
years plus a couple of months, he was *using his mind!*

I wish I could tell you that when Ben grew up, he was always so
eager to help, he maintained his desire to clean up the kitchen (and
even his room), and he had enough "smarts" to make it in this world
on his own. He didn't, of course, but then there are many of us who are
not always particularly helpful, neat, or self-sufficient.

What I can tell you is that Ben has accomplished what we came to expect of him and more—not at genius level, I grant you, but again, I never asked for that. All I asked for was to know—somehow—whether or not we had a child who could think, who would be able to appreciate, albeit in some ways limited, joys of the cognizant mind.

On a long-ago day I got my answer from a little boy who brought me a dust pan. His seemingly simple action seemed to me to be a promise of good things to come. And he has kept that promise.

# Finding the Holiday Spirit

. . . . . . . . . . . . . . . . . . . . . . . . . . . . . . . . . . . . . . . . . . . . . . . . . .

When Ben was six years old, he made the leap from nursery school to "real" school. Stephen Knolls, the school he landed in, was a public school serving mentally retarded students aged six to twenty-one. In the early 1970s, it was one of three such schools in Montgomery County, Maryland, where we live.

Ben had no trouble adjusting to Stephen Knolls; in fact, he liked it a lot. He already knew some of the kids through our parent group, and he quickly became fond of his teachers. There were about seven youngsters in this primary class, most of them kids with Down syndrome like Ben, and they were a lively bunch! It was in this class that first year that Ben learned to read.

Although Ben adapted quite well, *I* had a problem, and one which caused me considerable anguish and guilt. I'm not proud to admit this, but I found it very disturbing to see "older" kids with Down syndrome and older people with mental retardation in general. In fact, some of the students in their teens and twenties downright *scared* me when I thought in terms of the future. For one thing, I was bothered by their physical appearance. Some—particularly those with Down syndrome—were quite overweight. Others were extremely thin, and a few had very small heads and twisted limbs. Even more disquieting was how "out of it" many of the older students with Down syndrome appeared. They had a certain dullness of manner and facial expression that seemed so different from the high spirits that animated kids like Ben and his friends. I couldn't help wondering . . . . Someday would Ben be like this too? I knew these feelings were not unique with me. I had discussed them with other parents who admitted reacting the same way. But knowing I was in the same boat with others didn't make my feelings any more manageable.

When the notice came home that there would be a holiday program before Christmas vacation began and that all parents were invited, I was understandably apprehensive. Instead of just encountering one or two older students in the halls, I would be seeing *all* of them, more than I had ever seen at one time before. Frankly, I didn't know how I would handle it. But I was determined to go. Ben was so excited, I just couldn't let him down.

And so it was that on the Big Day I found myself in what looked like an ordinary auditorium in an ordinary school. I sat there with the dozens of other parents waiting for the holiday program to begin. I had attended more than my share of school programs, but I knew by the intrinsic nature of the school that this program would be different. But I didn't know what the "difference" would be.

The program began with the Primary Department, who came marching in decked out in green and red construction-paper collars and dressed in their very best. I tried to ignore the fact that the little kid in the front row singing so angelically and poking his pal in the ribs at the same time was *my* little kid.

Had "Jingle Bells" or "Jolly Old St. Nicholas" ever been sung with such fervor, and so off-key at the same time? Had "I Have a Little Dreidel" ever been danced with such gusto, such vigor, such foot-stamping enthusiasm? And, as the audience literally held its breath, had a piano solo of that same "Jingle Bells" ever been played with such determination, a slow-measured, two-fingered rendition carried through to its triumphant conclusion by a little girl who at first seemed about to run away? The heartfelt applause was returned with a very proper curtsey and a wide grin.

The Primary Department was followed by the Secondary Students and in turn by the Seniors, a few staff members interspersed among them. The boys were dressed in sports jackets and slacks, the girls in bright dresses. They looked terrific. But more than that, they had the look of "Can Do!" They were *involved*.

"Silver Bells" had been played to death in all the stores for weeks. But now I heard it as if for the first time, fresh and lilting and beautiful. And when I looked self-consciously around, I found that I was not alone. Others in the audience also had tears in their eyes and a tremor on their lips.

What was it about this simple school program which so stirred the hearts of those who came, and lifted up even the Scroogiest among us? Was it because most of us who attended that day were parents? Partly I suppose. But certainly that wasn't the whole reason. Maybe part of the response was because many of us were aware that not too many years ago, a lot of youngsters like these special kids of ours would not have been around for Christmas, for Hanukkah, for any holiday. Children like ours were kept in the dark corners of life. Not likely you'd see them at school, let alone participating in a holiday program.

And maybe that is why the enlightenment embodied in the music of this particular student body touched us all so deeply, and for me banished some of the apprehension and disturbing qualms which had so haunted me. As I watched those older students and listened to them sing, I couldn't help but think how lucky Ben and his peers were. As part of a new generation of children with mental retardation, they were already reaping the benefits of changed attitudes. When they got to be as old as those seniors, who knows what doors of opportunity might open for them?

On this note of hope I could rejoice. And what better time—what better place? Right there in that school auditorium, I got the lift to see me through. In an old-fashioned way it was finding the Holiday Spirit!

*I bet I'm not the only one who could hardly believe it when TV dramas began featuring characters with mental retardation who were actually shown as multi-faceted human beings. All of us, I think, feel an almost proprietary pride in gifted young actor Chris Burke, of "Life Goes On" fame. And Larry Drake's brilliant portrayal of Benny on "L.A. Law" has often hit home with painful reality. It's not just in drama, either, that we are seeing people with mental retardation in real-life settings. We are seeing them in TV commercials for products such as soap, toothpaste, food—not only in promos for Special Olympics. Let's not forget "Sesame Street," either, which was one of the first shows to include people with disabilities in its regular cast of characters. Viewers could actually see children with Down syndrome learning numbers and letters as other kids do!*

*Perhaps newer parents aren't that surprised and even take such programming for granted. But those of us who've been around for a while are still somewhat amazed and excited to see them; at least, I certainly am.*

*It's worth remembering, though, that until very recently there were inviolable taboos against showing kids with "something wrong"—particularly when that "something wrong" was mental retardation. And although some of the barriers have come down, I, for one, don't think individuals with disabilities are anywhere near as commonplace in commercials as they should be. I think the following essay, originally published in the Washington Star on April 27, 1981, gives a sense not only of how far we have come, but also of how far we have yet to go. At the time, it generated a number of letters to the editor all strongly agreeing with what I had to say. (Sadly, that fine old newspaper bit the dust a few months later after more than a hundred years of publishing.)*

# Those TV Commercials Are Passing Up a Natural

. . . . . . . . . . . . . . . . . . . . . . . . . . . . . . . . . . . . . . . . . .

Bumbling about the kitchen the other morning in my usual pre-breakfast fog, I managed to ask my young son which cereal he'd prefer. Let the record show that this kid will absolutely not eat a hot breakfast and wouldn't touch an egg if Super Chicken and Daffy Duck simultaneously appeared in person and laid one on his plate. So even if it makes me a less than perfect mother, I serve him what he will eat, cold cereal. The only question that begins each day is which kind of cold cereal.

He named his choice that morning with such gusto, such enthusiasm that I felt myself slipping into a TV commercial; the nurturing mother, the receptive/grateful child, and of course the perfect cereal. Ben is totally crazy (no pun intended) about the brand of cereal he chose that morning. Other kids get paid for saying what he was saying for free with sincere conviction.

But for all his sincerity, this young cereal lover of mine is the last child a manufacturer or advertising executive would use in a commercial. Children of TV commercials display many characteristics: cute, funny, bright, innocent, worldly wise, odd/appealing (What ever happened to Mason Reese?), but never . . . never mentally retarded.

Now, it is true that viewers do see mentally retarded children and persons with various handicaps on TV. We see them sometimes as part of dramatic productions, some very effective and moving dramas. And we often see them on appealing spots plugging various endeavors, the Special Olympics, for example. And we see "poster children" representing all kinds of disabling conditions. Almost always, if you think about it, these children appear with a celebrity, someone with a famous face who captures our attention, someone who most likely would be found on a baseball diamond, a golf course, a football field, a movie set—but almost certainly would not be found in an ordinary setting such as my kitchen.

The celebrity and the "Poster Child" are set apart, out of context. They appeal to our pocketbooks and our understanding via our emotions and the child is almost always presented as "special," which is OK, I suppose, and suited to the purpose of an appeal. But what does a "Poster Child" do in real life?

The children who dwell in the land of TV commercials are almost always shown in ordinary settings doing ordinary things. They gargle and brush their teeth, they put on bandages or pull them off with winsome ouches, they sell cool drinks from cleverly constructed "neighborhood stands," they steal pieces of mom's just-baked cake, they shampoo their dogs, they suffer with colds or warts and get instant relief with the proper product. And of course they eat cereal, just like my son.

Now let's get this straight. I am not a frustrated "movie mother"! I don't want my son in a TV commercial. My cat maybe, but not my kid. What I do want, however, is to see some kids like him on TV commercials. Commercials, exaggerated and obnoxious as they often are, use the milieu of daily life as their most common focal point in getting their message across. For many American families, daily life includes coping with, living with, and loving children who are mentally handicapped.

When we take a family trip our son goes too. If we were on TV trying out Dad's new "Radiant Rally Radials" or "Future Car" he would not be in that car with us.

When we bathe the family cats, all three of them, our son is there to help. If we were bathing cats on TV, or more likely a cute little Rover, with "Fleas Dead Forever" there'd be no helper like our son in the viewing picture.

When we celebrate Christmas, our family festivities focus a good bit on our son, partly because he is the youngest and he loves Christmas so much he makes it more meaningful for all of us. If we were gathered 'round the old TV Christmas Tree plugging toys and games, something our son knows a lot about, he'd never be shown at all.

A few years ago I wrote to the producer of a well-known soap opera and suggested a story line in which a family would have a retarded child. The producer took the time to answer me, but his response was totally negative. He said he was convinced that the idea of showing a family "suffering the heartbreak" of having a retarded child would be "too emotionally traumatic for the viewing audience." My first impulse, of course, was to write him back and tell him he was nuts and was underestimating the viewing public. Rape, incest, murder, blackmail;

those things are OK and don't upset people? But a loving child—a loving retarded child—would present emotional trauma?

Ah well, I learned a long time ago that where mental retardation is concerned it is better to save energy for battles that can be won and not expend it on fighting windmills.

However, it is interesting to note that several years after this disturbing correspondence a different soap opera did, in fact, present the exact problem which I had outlined, that of a family facing the possibility of having a retarded child. And a retarded youngster actually appeared in a number of episodes.

For the most part, the attitude of the producer to whom I wrote prevails in the world of TV commercials. No matter that like everybody else, retarded children and their families consume many of the products the junior pitch persons extol. The All American Family of TV commercials might be beset by many problems, from fleas on the dog to father's bleeding gums and mother's heart-breaking psoriasis, but one thing they've never had to worry about so far is an abnormal child. Eccentric maybe, normal surely.

Sometimes when I watch those delightful commercials featuring Bill Cosby—surely the best to be viewed—and I see those multi-hued, multi-ethnic, little charmers with him eating up their pudding with such natural joie de vivre, I long to see another kind of face there with them: a child or two, who like my son, is obviously mentally retarded, but who is also obviously a cherished and vital member of a viewing, consuming, "Typical American Family." He too eats pudding, uses band aids, needs children's aspirin, and has to fight cavities.

To those advertising geniuses who may recoil at the thought of a commercial showing a real-life kid who happens to be retarded, it's my guess that if you'll . . . *try* it . . . you'll *like* it . . . and so will the viewing public!

*And they do!*

*This article was first published in 1974, shortly before Public Law 94–142 was to open up a vast new arena of educational opportunities for children with disabilities. Our kids have made great progress since then, but I'm afraid I still couldn't answer the question in the title with an unqualified "yes." Could you?*

# Is the World Ready for the Graduates?

. . . . . . . . . . . . . . . . . . . . . . . . . . . . . . . . . . . .

L ast year I went to a graduation. As graduations go, it was a very small one. Five young people marched down the center aisle of the modest auditorium, flanked by seated families and friends. "Pomp and Circumstance" from the tape recorder evoked mood and memories. Baskets of flowers hung from the ceiling, their fragrance mingling with the warm evening air from the open doors and windows. Later that night, there would be spring showers.

I almost hadn't come at all. My throat was scratchy, I was tired, and, although my son was a primary student in the school, I didn't really know any of the graduates personally. But there I was, seated in the last row watching the four young men and one young woman solemnly make their way to the chairs set up for them in the front of the auditorium.

They turned to face us. The dignitaries awaiting them were sitting to their left. Except for the small size of the class and that instead of caps and gowns the boys were in slacks and sport jackets, the girl in a long dress, it looked much like any other graduation ceremony.

Like other graduations, it was sentimental and nostalgic, a fond look backward with tender recollections of the graduates as young children adjusting to their first days at school.

And, like other graduations, it was cognizant of the future, forward-looking and hopeful. The sheltering walls of school were to be left behind forever as the big world beckoned.

But for these graduates would the world, indeed, beckon?

The sense of accomplishment upon their graduation was obvious; the joy and pride showing plain on their faces. *They* were ready!

What about the rest of us?

The root word for *graduation* means step by step. The root word for *retarded* means slow. In a very real way the two words have a unique symbiosis, and nowhere is this better understood than at Stephen Knolls School, a public school in Montgomery County, Maryland, serving students with mental retardation *and* their families.

I went to this spring graduation at Stephen Knolls because it marked a milestone of achievement, not only for the students, but for all—parents, teachers, staff—who have loved and nurtured them.

It may be we should congratulate not only the graduates but ourselves as well. Less than twenty years ago there would have been no "Pomp and Circumstance" for these students, no proud parents assembled, no granting of diplomas. Less than twenty years ago there would have been no school like Stephen Knolls. As the popular slogan would have us believe, "We've come a long way. . . ."

Yet, sitting there watching those smiling faces at the graduation ceremony I wondered. How far have we *really* come? I wondered about those who have *not* loved and nurtured children such as ours, who have not known them at all.

I wondered about those who are automatically negative, or scared or indifferent. I wondered about those who are in utter ignorance about retardation, and remembered the jolt of despair I'd received from the woman in the drugstore who told her little boy to move away from mine because "his eyes look funny and you might catch it."

It was very easy to read the faces of the graduates. From my place in the last row I could not see the faces of their parents and friends. But I didn't have to see them to know that there were many there whose thoughts matched my own and who trembled at the bitter-sweetness we were witnessing.

Not too many years from now I'll be going to another graduation. In fact, the whole family will be going and we'll sit down front with other families of the graduates. Impossible as it is to visualize now, my son, that little kid who's so partial to field trips and so squirmy at the thought of homework, will be among the proud marchers.

There'll be the speeches and the diplomas and the congratulations. There'll be a look to the past and thoughts of the future. There'll be smiles and the music and the baskets of flowers.

And perhaps by then there'll hardly be anyone at all who cares if he has "funny eyes." And no one will want to move away from him. They'll just slow down a bit and walk with him.

*The year after I wrote this article, Ben and several of his classmates were mainstreamed into a regular elementary school. After P.L. 94–142 went into effect, mainstreaming became even more commonplace. In our county, one of the three schools for students with mental retardation was closed because of under-enrollment. Stephen Knolls was completely renovated and became a school for children with profound handicaps.*

*Every year we go back to Stephen Knolls for the school spring fair. Ben loves the games, meeting up with friends, and the food—oh those subs! He always enjoys seeing his old principal and former teachers, who greet him with warmth and affection. It's a great day! There are a lot of good memories in that school for Ben, and for all of us.*

*But it seems like a long time ago that he belonged there—if he ever did.*

# Phantoms

· · · · · · · · · · · · · · · · · · ·

**P**hantoms from my childhood have been haunting me lately, sad little shades who touched the fringes of my life.

One was a boy who would appear now and then in our neighborhood, nobody knew from where. A tall stringbean of a boy with ragged clothes way too tight, he always rode the same small, beat-up tricycle (*not* a bicycle), his knees sticking out at angles like some strange frog. He was probably about sixteen, a lot older than the rest of us. His name was Mickey, but half taunting, half in jest, we all called him "Ma-*Hick*-ey."

We knew nothing about him, not his full name, nor who his parents were, nothing, and we didn't much care. We only knew that we could tease him and get away with it.

He was "teched"—"not right in the head." The word *retarded* was not in our vocabulary. And if someone pulled him off his funny little tricycle and hid it, he'd cry, snuffling loudly and wiping at his eyes and nose. Some of the kids thought this was very funny and they'd roll the trike back and forth out of his reach, watching him blubber. Eventually, a few kids with consciences would retrieve it for him and he'd rub his eyes and grin, tears and dirt smearing his face.

It's a sure bet Mickey never went to school nor did much else. His life revolved around that little trike, and I can see him still, a ridiculous and pitiful figure pedaling up the block into nothingness.

The other phantom was a dark-haired, chunky girl with "funny eyes." We'd see her sitting on her front porch. If we stopped to look at her—*look*, not talk—her mother would immediately appear and lead her inside. We all knew why; the girl was a "Mongolian Idiot!"

Most of us past thirty probably have memories of similar "strange children" hovering at the edges of our lives. But rarely do we recall these children partaking of the same activities we did: school, movies on a Saturday afternoon, circuses, ballets, picnics, swimming, ice skating—the mundane, sometimes not so mundane, events of everyday life.

New parents of children with handicaps must find it almost impossible to believe that in the not too distant past, children like ours were a nearly invisible population with few rights to anything, certainly not a right to be educated. Today it is taken for granted that our children with Down syndrome will go to early intervention, preschool, *school*. It is the *norm*. But it did not begin to become the norm until 1975. That year, Congress—prodded by parent advocacy—passed a new federal law, Public Law 94–142, declaring that every child has a right to a public school education *no matter the handicap*. Until then, parents and teachers "ahead of their time" had been teaching youngsters with mental retardation for years and knew their capabilities. But there was no overall commitment to the idea of education for the mentally handicapped.

Other laws have followed Public Law 94–142. Laws are now on the books affirming the right to work, right to patronize public establishments, right to use public transportation, right not to be discriminated against—rights which "normal" people barely think about in the course of their daily activities, and certainly not in terms of *law* and *rights*. We go about the business of living so automatically. In time, people with handicaps may go about it automatically too.

Yes, things have changed dramatically for the better since "the good old days" when many of us were growing up. We have only to look around to know that this is so.

Today the general public is getting used to seeing people with mental retardation in many areas of society. Kids with mental retardation are often in regular schools, and superb actors who actually have mental retardation appear on TV programs. Special Olympics has moving and realistic commercials, and we are even seeing regular commercials which include people with mental retardation. More and more people with mental retardation are showing up in the work place, our own kids among them. We can feel pretty good about changing attitudes, and I do.

But sometimes I get wary, and with good reason, I believe.

Almost every year, for as long as I can remember, the Washington, D.C.-area media has carried stories, *awful* stories, which forcefully remind me that enlightened attitudes about mental retardation don't reign quite everywhere yet. These stories are about a local residential facility for people with mental retardation. This particular facility was supposed to have been phased out and closed forever years ago, but somehow this has never happened. Year after year the media does its annual expose, and everybody gets terribly upset and demands action, and then the story fades until next time. The pictures, which are particularly graphic on TV, show "residents" sitting on the floor doing nothing, up against a wall banging their heads, curled motionless on a bed, wandering down corridors screeching, or standing quietly waiting for someone—anyone—who never comes.

Of course, there are always the obligatory scenes of filthy bathrooms and stark "recreation areas," followed by interviews with officials who explain about the shortage of help, constant turnover of staff, resistance in neighborhoods to the group homes where the "residents" are supposed to go once the facility is closed, and always, always *lack of funding*.

This Home for the Retarded reflecting the ignorance, neglect, and cruelty of an era supposed to be gone forever exists under the very noses of people *we* elected (elected from every state in the Union, don't forget). And make no mistake, every politician and government official residing in the Washington, D.C., area is aware of this infamous facility.

I'm not making a political statement *per se*. I am really expressing an observation, and a conclusion. If we—all of us—are not ever aware, ever questioning, ever skeptical, the future well-being of *our* kids is in jeopardy, no doubt about it. I'm convinced of this because each time stories about this facility surface, it is hard to escape the fact that the "residents" of the "home" are overwhelmingly poor. Most have no one to speak up for them; no dedicated, savvy, mad-as-hell, articulate parents, no one with any kind of power of persuasion to get something done. The media does its job of showing the awful truth, and a lot of people say "Tch, tch!" But when all the sound and fury subsides, where are those who are truly involved and committed? Where are those who could make something happen for the absolutely helpless, powerless "residents" of a "home" which is no home at all?

If we are under the impression that politicians, property owners, institutional officials, and others who have a vested interest in keeping intact the power structure of an institution are going to do anything out of the simple goodness of their hearts for kids like ours, we've been seeing too many happy-ending movies. Call me a cynic, but I believe this to be true.

There *is* much good going on these days on behalf of people with mental retardation, and all handicaps; we have only to look at what has happened and continues to happen with education, jobs, community involvement, and public awareness. Certainly we *do* live in a more enlightened time than times gone by. I'm not denying it. Rather, I am saying that we must be vigilant and guard what has been gained. It is, in fact, this very enlightenment which defines the horror of the place supported by the government of our nation's capital. Ironic that part of its name is "haven." I suspect there are other such "havens" throughout our country, more than we care to know about. And a question we have to ask ourselves is *why?* Why do we let them continue to exist?

When I ask that question, a faint echo of memory—the phantoms—seems to touch me. Even as kids on our block long ago, we could see that nobody much cared about the future of "Ma-*Hickey*" and the dark-haired little girl. We could figure out that "dummies" were good for teasing and interesting to stare at, even if it kind of gave you the creeps. We could tease and stare with impunity; who'd stick up for *them?* Of course, we were awfully glad that whatever had happened to them hadn't happened to us. But we didn't dwell on it much. We were too busy going to school, having fun, doing all the things normal kids do. And when we all grew up and went away, those two were out of our lives forever. What became of them had nothing to do with us.

I'd like to think that Mickey and the girl ended up okay, but almost surely they didn't. More likely, they wound up in a "haven" waiting . . . just waiting for someone to come.

# It's Not Funny, But. . . .

. . . . . . . . . . . . . . . . . . . . . . . . . . . . . . . . . . . . . . . . . . . . . . . . .

Years ago when Ben was born with Down syndrome, a friend said, "If it had to happen to any of us, it's probably better that it happened to the two of you." I didn't understand those words at the time, although I knew they were spoken with love and concern, and I'm not sure I understand them today.

But I think I have learned from them.

Back then I cried a lot. The pain was fresh and new—something was wrong with our beautiful baby and nothing would ever be right again. Certainly words were no help, especially words that were a puzzlement. Better to say nothing at all.

Well, as the old adage goes, a lot of water has flowed under the bridge since then. And like many members of the Montgomery County Association for Retarded Citizens, we have gone from being among the "walking wounded" to wanting to reach out and lend a helping hand to others.

It's easy enough to give people information about programs, schooling, agencies, etc. But how do you make the mother or father of a brand new baby with Down syndrome believe that some day they will smile—even laugh—again? That they will want to see a movie, go to the beach, take the baby to the zoo? That they will ever stop focusing on this overwhelming problem and actually enjoy life again?

One thing I avoid at all costs is waxing philosophic. These parents may or may not have a philosophy of their own to help them through, but they will never hear from me that it's meant to be; better you than your cousin; it's part of a plan we don't understand, etc. Platitudes, no matter how heartfelt, are so offensive to me that I simply cannot inflict them on frightened and confused parents.

What then? How can you help people you don't really know, yet whose pain you understand only too well?

First of all, you listen. You let them talk and you just listen; you are there.

And then, it seems to me, you must touch them with humor, however gently. You must find a way to make them smile. If they can smile today, no matter how small or tremulous that smile may be, then deep down they'll be aware that the time will come when the smile will be bigger. And if a smile, why not someday a laugh?

Please understand, I'm not for a minute advocating that we sock new parents with a big production number that "this is a barrel of laughs and you don't know what you've been missing up to now." We're not attempting a new version here of "Laugh In."

There is nothing funny about having a retarded child. But the fact remains that sometimes that child does funny things, and if we can't laugh about it life has, indeed, lost its zest.

Consider the Great Socks On-Going Caper, enough to drive any reasonable parent (include teachers, especially gym teachers) crazy, and yet. . . .

What do you do about a kid who insists on wearing seven pairs of sweat socks at the same time, with sneakers yet? You can talk until your jaw aches about appropriate behavior, time lost peeling socks on and off, the disadvantages of constricted toes (talk about smelly feet!). You can resort to removing the socks from his dresser and hiding them, knowing full well that eventually he will find them and that you will see him one morning running to catch the school bus, his legs looking like swaddled hams and too late for you to do a thing about it.

I think that most of us would agree that pride and panic often vie for space in the hearts of those of us who have retarded children. How can we not cheer them when we see them using their abilities, their perceptions, their intelligence? Ah, sweet memories to cherish of positive genius manifesting itself at the wrong time in the wrong place.

Like most kids today, Ben has friends of various ethnic backgrounds, and he knows about the countries they or their parents have come from. Having friends from other parts of the world is a normal aspect of life.

But oh the impact of television and the late Bruce Lee!

One afternoon I had taken Ben with me when I went to get a haircut and shampoo. Imagine the trapped feeling of sitting under a hair dryer at your favorite beauty parlor and seeing your child suddenly rise and go into a Kung Fu routine because he recognizes that the young man entering for a haircut has Asian features. Oh boy!

It was plain to see that the poor fellow had no idea why this strange kid was leaping about him in such bizarre fashion, but I did and I shrank back against my chair, wishing fervently that the hair dryer would malfunction, blow up, set my hair on fire—anything to cause a distraction.

Suffice it to say we left with my hair still wet, and Ben got the lecture of his life on appropriate behavior, inappropriate behavior, no-good-lousy behavior, no candy-no-ice-cream-no-pizza-no-TV behavior.

But I have to confess, when I conjure up that scene in my mind I find myself grinning.

Now and again I wonder how it might have been had Ben been normal. We all do this, don't we? How different the texture of his life and ours would have been. Different, but—I'm convinced—not necessarily more challenging.

Of course, there are challenges and challenges. There is no one in this world who can set me up for one better than Ben Trainer. I am the oldest member of our local swimming pool to have jumped—make that doddered—off the diving board, because Ben said if I did it he would too, and then he chickened out.

Ben's challenges have a way of catching me off guard. Picture this scene, if you will. I'm standing in the hall putting towels away in the linen closet. Ben and his great chum, Laura, having finished their after-school-before-Special-Olympics snack, are in Ben's room, door ajar, playing records. And then those magic words, "Let's play doctor."

The big "It"! I remind myself to remain calm as I pick up the towels which now cover my feet. I will handle this with tact, nonchalance. Certainly no scolding, no reproach. Cool and rational, that will be me. Ready to answer any tricky question, open up a great discussion.

I step into the room trying to look exceptionally pleasant. Laura is stretched out on the bed, her mouth open as wide as a mouth can be, and Ben is bending over her meticulously counting her teeth, one by one, with her tongue and tonsils thrown in for good measure.

Sweet relief! It's Doctor of Dentistry they're playing!

"If it had to happen to any of us, it's probably better that it happened to the two of you." Those enigmatic words of long ago; they don't come to mind too often anymore.

There are other things to think of . . . and often laugh about.

*We never know when or how these kids of ours will strike a spark in us that will, as the old song goes, light up our lives. Usually it seems to be something rather ordinary that somehow turns into something illuminating. This is what happened to me one day when Ben was about eight years old, and I ended up writing this essay.*

# He's Lucky, This Little Boy

· · · · · · · · · · · · · · · · · · · · · · · · · · · · · · · · · · · · · · · · · · · · · · · · · · · ·

If this turns out to be Pollyanna-like I hope no one reads it, or else reads it and writes a nasty letter. Being a Pollyanna can be tolerated in some instances I suppose, but never in regard to mental retardation. And that's what this is about, mental retardation, or more precisely, certain feelings I have toward my son who is mentally retarded.

Now believe me, I have had my moments of weeping and despair. When I first learned that our baby, that rosy, dimpled infant, was retarded I almost died of agony. The doctors were wrong. Ben—we'd named him in part for Bennett Cerf whom we didn't know but had long admired—our Ben couldn't be what they said, a child with Down syndrome.

But he was and he is, and that's a primary fact of his life and ours.

Today Ben is a sturdy eight-year-old. And if sometimes I find tears in my eyes at the sight of him trying so hard to keep up with his neighborhood peers who are so brightly normal, I more often find myself smiling, sometimes even belly laughing, at the sheer exuberance with which this child faces life.

The very idea for writing this at all is that not an hour ago I witnessed the most ecstatic, uninhibited reaction to a fried-chicken TV commercial that any sponsor could not hope for in his wildest dreams.

Who else can raise his arms in gustatory triumph over a dancing chicken and shout "Wow!" in such a way as Ben: What an ability to translate the mundane into something terrific! It gives his life an added flavor at every turn.

He is lucky, this little boy of mine. He will not conquer the worlds of the academic, the scientific, or the great doers. But he has a unique appreciation for those ordinary rites of life that seem only dull and jaded to the rest of us.

And it goes way beyond fried chicken.

The neighbors' dog comes loping by covered with mud from a nearby creek and all we see is one big messy mutt. But Ben sees a friend, and they sit on the walk together, Ben's arm around dog's neck, dog licking Ben's face; sheer joy in one another.

We go to the ocean and contemplate its vast magnificence. The ocean fills a hole Ben has dug in the sand. "Beat it, Ocean," says Ben.

Around 3:20 every afternoon the front door bangs open and various articles are dropped on the floor. "I'm back, Mommy!" shouts Ben and comes to give me my home-again hug.

One recent Saturday morning the whole family had slept late, and as my husband and I were struggling awake Ben came into our room to say good morning. He looked at his stubble-chinned, disheveled father and in the tone of a true believer announced, "Daddy is Prince Charming."

At that moment I could see more of a resemblance to Godzilla, but Ben saw Prince Charming. And then he turned to me—a half-unconscious Phyllis Diller—and said, "Mommy is the Sleeping Beauty!"

How wonderful to wake to laughter. And how wonderful to live with someone who can look at a couple of creaky parents and see a prince and princess.

Pollyanna, go fly a kite.

But Ben Trainer, oh how I love you!

# Diary Excerpts

. . . . . . . . . . . . . . . . . . . . . . . . . . . . .

For many years I have kept a diary, just a few lines jotted down at the end of each day. There is nothing profound in my notations, no earth-shattering pronouncements. It's a simple record of events and feelings that mean something to me. Because I use small, five-year diaries with only enough space for about five lines per date, through the years I have learned to be very economical in my words. The events of each day are scribbled quickly with no thought about repetition, artistic content, or in-depth analysis. If I've written almost the same thing the day before, so what? Many days of a stay-at-home mom are alike. Besides, no one has ever read my diaries, and I certainly never intended that anyone would!

Every now and then, I go back and look at what I wrote in past years. For example, I sometimes do this as Ben's birthday approaches. Recently, I pulled out the one which chronicled the year of Ben's birth. At that time, Allen and I had been married almost thirteen years. Douglas was close to ten, Ann was about to turn eight, and Claire was four and a half. We had thought our family was complete!

As I read through the pages, I realized that here was a unique opportunity to share the wrenching emotions at the very time I was experiencing them, from the early floundering days after Ben's diagnosis through a period which brought significant changes to a family, and—probably most of all—to the mother in that family: me. Here too was a chance to let other parents see that no matter how much a diagnosis of Down syndrome may consume you today, eventually the focus of your life shifts and you get on with your life—and in ways you never expected. I think the words I set down so long ago will be meaningful to anyone who has had a baby born "less than perfect."

Here, then, are excerpts from my diary written during the first three years of Ben's life.

# Year One

Went into labor this morning . . . and Baby Ben [Bennett] was born to us at 3:28 p.m.

. . . . . . .

Groggy . . . Baby looks like Allen and Douglas. He is not too strong in his grip. Very placid and contented. I do love holding him . . . he's so small.

. . . . . . .

Dr. Snow says that the baby's muscles are lacking in tone. . . . She wants some tests made. He is so cute and cuddly. I'm so worried.

. . . . . . .

They took the baby away today to Children's Hospital. It was an awful thing to go through. This could be very serious. I'm sick.

. . . . . . .

They let me come home. I was climbing walls. Annie is brokenhearted because the baby didn't come home. It may take three weeks.

. . . . . . .

Allen went to work . . . came home at noon to feed me. We didn't hear a word about the baby. I feel so hopeless.

. . . . . . .

My milk is drying up. I'm sick about it. I called the nursery today and heard the babies crying and I cried and cried. But Allen talked to the doctor and she said the baby is responding and doing well. . . . Oh, I hope so.

. . . . . . .

Allen and I went down to see the baby today. He certainly seems livelier . . . hard to believe . . . I just hope he will be okay . . . it all seems like a dream.

. . . . . . .

The baby—our baby—is a Mongoloid. We were told today. . . . Allen knew, poor darling. I guess I was suspicious . . . but I'm in shock.

. . . . . . .

I just feel so tired. When I think how scared I was all through pregnancy about this very thing. Allen is so mature about it.

. . . . . . .

I am so tired, so tired. I'm all right when I talk with Allen but when I'm alone and start thinking I get panic stricken. If we could only go back.

. . . . . . .

Mom and Dad called. We've decided not to tell them. They're not well.

. . . . . . .

Lynn [a long-time friend] came by and I told her. . . . I still can't believe it and I think in a way my heart will break. It's so unfair it's beyond belief. I felt so sad today. I just can't believe it and I fear the years of responsibility. . . . If I could only go back.

. . . . . . .

We brought the baby home. The kids are so excited. I'm in a daze. He seems lively . . . but I wish we had never had another one. I'm awful.

. . . . . . .

The baby was good last night . . . he's really very good . . . but it's not the same. I'm just wounded.

. . . . . . .

The baby is so cute but when I think of the future?

. . . . . . .

I'm depressed. Poor little Ben. I can see his little face will be flat looking when he's older. He's so cute right now. It breaks my heart. I hate God!

. . . . . . .

Baby was good today but I'm so tired tonight and I still have to feed him. It does no good to look back but I feel so bitter. It shouldn't be this way.

. . . . . . .

Easter Sunday . . . big deal. It was a pretty day, though. If only Ben would really smile at me. I wish I didn't feel so bitter.

. . . . . . .

Ann's birthday party. Shawn swallowed part of a plastic spoon. Haven't heard yet how she is.

. . . . . . .

Ben smiled today. He's cute. I just don't know what to think.

. . . . . . .

We went down to the Mall this morning to the Transportation Exhibit, baby too. It was fun. Nine weeks ago tomorrow he was born. He's smiling.

. . . . . . .

I cleaned and made formula wrong, I think. I was bitter today thinking about things. I just don't know if I'm adjusted.

. . . . . . .

Baby smiled a lot today. He is so cute. I just wonder if he has a real future.

. . . . . . .

I registered Claire for kindergarten. . . . Ben started solid food and loves it! He is cute . . . and very appealing.

. . . . . . .

It was more peaceful today but I'm always tense. Ben is so cute . . . sure loves his carrots and cereal.

. . . . . . .

We drove Grandma up home [to Allentown, Pennsylvania] and back in one day. The kids were obnoxious . . . Ben was good . . . but the others in the car, ugh.

. . . . . . .

I was so tired today I didn't do anything. When I think of a year ago I keep wanting to go back and make everything come out right.

. . . . . . .

Took Ben to Dr. Snow for his checkup. He's doing fine, apparently. Ben's a thumb sucker.

. . . . . . .

School's out. First day of vacation and Ann poked her hand though the glass door and had to have five stitches. Ye gods!

. . . . . . .

The Sheas had the nicest cookout. We all went. Ben was so good, he really is the best baby. It was so good to socialize.

. . . . . . .

We all ended up on the beach today, even Ben. He is so good! If only it had been warmer.

. . . . . . .

Ben is six months old today. Boy, does it make me think.

. . . . . . .

I must say Ben is awfully cute and loving. He's really very sweet.

. . . . . . .

. . . Gave Ben two baths . . . he loves it.

. . . . . . .

I felt depressed today . . . seeing pictures of some retarded children. Ben does look very mongoloid at times.

. . . . . . .

I felt so tired today. . . . Ben is getting so cute and lively!

. . . . . . .

Last night Allen and I watched a program about a Mongoloid child. I saw it last year when I was PG. It was sad but inspiring in some ways.

. . . . . . .

We all watched "The Great Pumpkin." Ben is so cute tonight.

. . . . . . .

Ben is nine months old. It doesn't seem possible.

. . . . . . .

Ben sort of crawled today. He sure is cute and lively.

. . . . . . .

We went on a train excursion to Harper's Ferry; it was fun. . . . Ben was so good. The kids loved it too.

. . . . . . .

I went up to the Plaza today shopping with Claire and Ben and ended up bringing home a stray dog . . . the dog howled all night.

. . . . . . .

Ben has a cold but he is so cute and lively tonight.

. . . . . . .

Ben is ten months old. He sure is cute.

. . . . . . .

December 31st. Snowed all day! Gee—I remember a year ago so well. [The year] went so fast. I can't believe all that's happened.

. . . . . . .

# Year Two

I keep thinking of last year, how did I know something was wrong? I seemed to know all along. Ben is a little under the weather.

. . . . . . .

Ben's got a jump seat. . . . It's snowy and cold. Ben was so cute today. He likes his jump seat.

. . . . . . .

Ben got on his hands and knees a lot. . . . Took him to Dr. Snow for a checkup. He's over sixteen pounds.

. . . . . . .

I'll never forget a year ago today if I live to be 100. [The day Ben was taken to Children's Hospital supposedly for half a day and ended up staying a month.]

. . . . . . .

Mom called today. . . . I'll never tell her the truth.

. . . . . . .

Teachers on strike . . . the kids were all home. House is a mess.

. . . . . . .

Kids still home. Ben was so cute and lively today.

. . . . . . .

Ann thinks she has poison on her hands and is crying and crying.

. . . . . . .

Went to dinner at Sheas but Ben made such a fuss with the sitter we had to come home.

. . . . . . .

Went to Dr. Harmon for my checkup. He thought Ben looked great. Went to Sandy Spring Firehouse for dinner. Fun!

. . . . . . .

Gee—one year ago [we brought Ben home]. Ben was so cute today.

. . . . . . .

Ben is wheezy but sweet. Claire is getting better but pale.

. . . . . . .

Went to Giffords [ice cream parlor]. Ben had his own ice cream.

. . . . . . .

I strolled Ben today. He liked it. He's awfully cute.

. . . . . . .

A pretty day. Ben will stand up in his jump seat when we tell him and he shakes hands. He's becoming more of a little boy.

. . . . . . .

Mom called. Dad's in the hospital.

. . . . . . .

We planted things. I'm trying to grow a lawn. . . . I sort of like gardening.

. . . . . . .

We got a kitten today. . . . Ben seems to be doing a little more. He waves a lot . . . so cute . . . so cute and sweet.

. . . . . . .

I bought a cute bathing suit today, hope it's not too young. I strolled Ben this afternoon.

. . . . . . .

We drove up to The Strasburg [train] today. . . . Ben is so good and enjoyed it.

. . . . . . .

The cat wet on Ann's bed—got to train her.

. . . . . . .

My birthday . . . Allen and the kids and I went to the buffeteria for dinner, came home, and had cake and presents. It was fun and nice.

. . . . . . .

Well, the dryer is broken today and spewing gas. I'm a wreck!

. . . . . . .

Ben is starting to sit up. He sure is cute. . . . We ordered a new dryer, the old one broke down again.

. . . . . . .

Ben is trying to say "Friskie" [the dog's name]. He is so cute.

. . . . . . .

Ben's first little tooth popped through today.

. . . . . . .

Bought Ben a little pool and a swing.

. . . . . . .

We put Ben in his little pool. He had a good time. He sits up so straight.

. . . . . . .

Ben went in his pool; he loves it!

. . . . . . .

Ben is sitting very well. He stands in the playpen too.

. . . . . . .

Ben looked so cute today. He's standing more and more . . . a rascal!

. . . . . . .

Mom called; Daddy's in the hospital. [My father died shortly after I made this entry; Allen's mother and my mother died a few months later. In fact, my mother died only six weeks before she was to take a much-anticipated visit to see Ben for the first time. I have chosen not to include the diary entries which focused on these wrenching losses.]

. . . . . . .

Took Ben and went up to the Plaza and bought some shoes. . . . Ben is a good little kid.

. . . . . . .

Ben is heavy to lift and so wiggly.

. . . . . . .

Trick or Treat. I went out too in a sheet.

. . . . . . .

I was at the polls all [election] day, the kids too, for the school board . . . am beat tonight . . . fun, though.

. . . . . . .

Ben is crawling on his hands and knees and almost standing without pulling up.

. . . . . . .

Ben seems to be on the verge of standing alone. He is crawling on all fours too. Claire can read!

. . . . . . .

The psychiatrist came to visit Ben. He said I was doing a great job with Ben, that his personality was very developed. It was gratifying.

. . . . . . .

It snowed today. . . . Ben loves to get into everything. . . . He's so busy.

. . . . . . .

Ben is able to stand alone if he wants to. He sure is cute, I must say, and quite alert. Into everything!

. . . . . . .

Ben's doing the elephant walk!

. . . . . . .

Ben is 23 months today. We went to a party . . . a very nice party, good to get out.

. . . . . . .

We are just staying home tonight. The house is a horrible mess. It doesn't seem like New Year's . . . can't believe this year is over.

. . . . . . .

# Year Three

When we ask Ben how old he is he says "two" (sort of). . . . I started an article about Ben today. It's been on my mind but I don't know if it will do. . . .

. . . . . . .

Gee, how I wish my article would sell. I need to express myself so much. . . . Ugh, Claire threw up tonight, she's very pale.

. . . . . . .

Had dinner at Anchor Inn . . . good to get out. Douglas did the baby sitting!

. . . . . . .

Annie threw up last night, has a fever today.

. . . . . . .

Ann's got a temperature. Claire's got a temperature and Ben threw up.

. . . . . . .

Ben was so listless this morning but seems better tonight. . . . He's so sweet.

. . . . . . .

A sad day. Daisy [the cat] was run over and killed this morning. We are all sick over it. The poor kids.

. . . . . . .

We adopted another cat [found in a tree], pregnant at that!

. . . . . . .

Ben is taking steps alone now. . . . He has bronchitis.

. . . . . . .

I got Ben's hair cut, what a fuss! He looks so cute, so much like Doug at his age.

. . . . . . .

Ben is two years old. We had a birthday cake and ice cream and presents. He was so cute!

. . . . . . .

Ben is taking steps alone, then he plops down. He's so funny.

. . . . . . .

*Redbook* sent back my article on Ben and I'm so disappointed.

. . . . . . .

I called Mom and talked a long time. She has no idea about Ben. . . . She's going into the hospital for tests.

. . . . . . .

Took Ann for ballet slippers. Made pea soup. Ben is into everything.

. . . . . . .

Ben is walking more every day. He's so cute and loving.

. . . . . . .

Took the kids to Wheaton Regional Park. . . . Ben enjoys it so much.

. . . . . . .

Diane [the cat] had her kittens last night in our bedroom, five cute little tigers. The kids all watched.

. . . . . . .

Took Ben to NIH [National Institutes of Health] to a speech therapist. It was very interesting and informative. Ben did well, I think. Allen and I went to PTA. I'm pooped.

. . . . . . .

A letter from Mom, she can't come in May, she's not well enough. I do wonder if I'll ever see her again.

. . . . . . .

We are planning a dinner party next week. I hope I know what I'm doing. Ben is darling!

. . . . . . .

The cat messed in our room again and wrecked our bedspread. I'm so damn mad!

. . . . . . .

Doug is twelve years old. My little baby.

. . . . . . .

A lovely spring day. I moved cat and kittens to the tool shed.

. . . . . . .

The kittens are so cute. . . . Ben loves being outside. He gets so dirty.

. . . . . . .

Ben and I went up and watched Ann and Claire at their dancing lessons. He liked it.

. . . . . . .

Took the kids to dinner . . . Hot Shoppe . . . even Ben, he was so good and ate so much!

. . . . . . .

Am trying to find homes for the kittens. . . . I've called everyone I can think of. . . .

. . . . . . .

Whew, a hectic day. I even played baseball in the street.

. . . . . . .

We joined Parkland pool today . . . haven't been swimming yet.

. . . . . . .

Took the kids to the pool for the first time. I think it will be nice. Ben enjoyed it.

. . . . . . .

Ben is so cute. . . . He plays with a doll.

. . . . . . .

Ben did the cutest, smartest thing. He got the dust pan for me when I was sweeping.

. . . . . . .

What a surprise! *Baby Talk Magazine* has accepted my article on Ben for $50.

. . . . . . .

Took the kids swimming. I do love to swim . . . get tired chasing Ben.

. . . . . . .

I've got an idea for a book about Ben, it's just formulating but it might go.

. . . . . . .

Made it up to Cacapon and to the cabin. Ben loves the sand on the beach.

. . . . . . .

I wrote letters to senators today . . . about fund cutting of medical research [into Down syndrome].

. . . . . . .

I've been typing letters like mad.

. . . . . . .

Dr. Coleman's secretary called and is sending a list of people for me to call about writing letters on behalf of research.

. . . . . . .

I've been making calls all day . . . a great response. . . . I've talked to some nice mothers. . . .

. . . . . . .

Went to see a young mother who lives near here . . . went to Virginia to pick up some pamphlets for mailing.

. . . . . . .

Got off more letters today.

. . . . . . .

Trying Ben on puzzles.

. . . . . . .

The *Post* and the *Star* had big articles on Dr. Coleman's research, very exciting.

. . . . . . .

Drove over to see an English train, the Scotsman, go down the track.

. . . . . . .

Allen and I are both working on ways to help get funds for the [research] program.

. . . . . . .

Ann took Ben Trick or Treating.

. . . . . . .

Allen and I and other parents had a meeting with an NIH doctor . . . an overall money shortage. . . .

. . . . . . .

We went over to the Wyman's in Virginia for a meeting about organizing "Mothers of Young Mongoloids." I don't know what to think.

. . . . . . .

I'm planning a "coffee" here for the mothers.

, , . . . . . .

The "coffee" went very well. Had a long-distance call from a woman in New York who wants to meet with us.

. . . . . . .

I had a letter in the *Washington Post* today . . . about the research. It's a good letter.

. . . . . . .

Got a call today from some congressman's office to tell me he's putting my letter in *The Congressional Record*.

. . . . . . .

A poor young mother called who saw my letter.

. . . . . . .

Both Doug and Claire threw up last night.

. . . . . . .

A reporter from *The Sentinel* called me today. I think there'll be a story on Thursday [about the Down syndrome research]. I'm so tired.

. . . . . . .

Doug and I baked pumpkin pie tonight. I talked to another reporter from a TV station.

. . . . . . .

Allen and I delivered some material to a TV station. Senator Tydings is appealing to Congress to restore funds to HEW.

. . . . . . .

A woman from Charles County called me—she'd seen my letter in the *Post*. . . . I hope things will simmer down after this week, I'm beat.

. . . . . . .

Whew! What an exciting day, we all went down to Congress [for hearings on funding for research; our letter-writing campaign paid off]. I think it went very well.

. . . . . . .

Well, they came and taped us [at our home], the TV crew, and it was fun and interesting.

. . . . . . .

My letter was in the *Star* tonight.

. . . . . . .

Claire became a Brownie! She's so cute and proud. We all went to Chinese dinner tonight. . . . Ben enjoyed it tremendously!

. . . . . . .

Had a nice letter from Representative Gude commending me for my letter in the *Post*.

. . . . . . .

We had a meeting here tonight and I think we're setting up a foundation.

. . . . . . .

Wrote more letters. How did I ever get into all this?

. . . . . . .

Congress reconvened today.

. . . . . . .

HEW bill vetoed.

. . . . . . .

Ben is three . . . so cute . . . it's hard to believe. . . .

. . . . . . .

# The Dream

. . . . . . . . . . . . . . . . . . . . . . . .

Shortly after we brought Ben home from the hospital for the first time, I began to have a recurring dream. In truth it was more than a dream; it was a nightmare of awful intensity. It so disturbed me that I became afraid to go to sleep.

The nightmare was always the same. I was somewhere outdoors in a wide expanse of open space. Close against me I was cradling a small, fragile baby rabbit. Above us swirled a huge, black, cape-like cloud which in some way meant terrible peril for the little rabbit. Without understanding how or why, I knew that I was the one who must keep the black cape-cloud from destroying the helpless little creature that somehow now belonged to me. In the world of my dream I was running and running, desperately looking for a hiding place, and the cloud effortlessly followed us, always hovering above, waiting to envelope the rabbit, and me too. I knew that the cloud was a powerful force—God turned cruel and evil, Fate, call it what you will—and as fast as I ran, I could not escape it. Both of us, the tiny rabbit and I, were helpless and could do nothing to elude that terrifying cloud. Even after I awoke, gasping and sobbing, the terror lingered on.

Usually I steer clear of dream interpretation. But I do think this particular dream had a pretty obvious meaning. The baby rabbit was, of course, Ben. And the sense of overwhelming responsibility with no *way out*, thrust upon me by a force beyond my control, was frighteningly real and left me feeling as helpless as my imperiled baby bunny.

I suspect that this kind of dream is very common to parents who've just found out that their baby has a disability. In fact, a national magazine recently ran a story about a young Hollywood actress who had a similar dream for weeks following the birth of a baby with severe disabilities, a baby who eventually died.

After all these years, I can still vividly recall the two feelings in my dream of unmitigated *responsibility* and *helplessness*. In or out of the dream, I feared facing them. I'm sure, in fact, that these feelings triggered the dream. I *did not want* to be *responsible* for this little creature—bunny or baby. And, unprepared, on the brink of despair, I felt *helpless* to do anything for something or someone even more helpless than I.

No wonder I was afraid to go to sleep at night. Eventually I came to terms with the meaning of my dream, the dream faded, and I was able to sleep again.

The *responsibility* has been awesome, no denying that. But it's also been the ultimate challenge of our lives and one which has brought a joy we could not have expected.

The *helplessness*—so feared—proved to be ephemeral. Simply put, we could not afford to be helpless if we wanted Ben to have a full and useful life. We could not afford to let Ben be helpless either.

I've had many dreams; few that I remember. Yet I cannot forget that small baby rabbit and the panicky fear which consumed me as I searched in vain for safety. It all seemed so unbearably real.

But it was only a dream.

# Myths and Images

. . . . . . . . . . . . . . . . . . . . . . . . . . . . . . . .

When Ben returns from his two weeks of summer camp each year, he always brings back what can best be described as "Laundry from Hell." After all these years I ought to be used to it, but I'm still in awe of what those clothes look like as I chuck them into the washer.

The first time Ben went off to camp, he was about nine or ten. The counselors sent a specific list of what to pack and we followed it to the letter. On the day we drove him up to camp, we wanted him to make a good impression, to look like the perfect young camper. I have a snapshot taken of him that day standing beside the car just before we said a teary goodbye. (Well, I was teary, at any rate.)

There he is, impeccable haircut, new blue tank-top shirt, matching blue shorts, white socks trimmed in blue, new red sneakers. He looks absolutely smashing—like a child model from the Sear's catalog.

Two weeks later he returned home a swamp creature. Little Boy Blue was gone, to be seen never more, except in his snapshot. A bug-bitten, scratching, shaggy-haired kid partial to dirt had replaced him. His trunk with the mud-encrusted clothes (and what else we could only guess) went straight to the laundry room. Despite what the detergent commercials promise, the coordinated blue outfit was never the same again. Nor was our perception of what makes a successful camper.

As the parent of a child with mental retardation, I find myself thinking about perceptions a lot. There are relatively harmless perceptions, such as my own image of the "happy camper." But there are others that can do grave damage by setting our children apart and creating unrealistic expectations for them.

As recently as twenty years ago, there was the old myth that babies with Down syndrome were hopeless "Mongoloids"—or worse yet, "Mongolian Idiots." The terms conjured up images which drove parents into instant grief and despair. And we know about the self-fulfilling prophecies which often doomed those so labeled to back rooms, institutions, or at the very least, to no education. Today it seems as if we have gone from the myth of the hopeless Mongoloid to another myth—a sort of deification.

Allen and I are by nature reasonably polite and we care about other people's feelings and sensibilities. But what about our own? How many times have we winced inwardly, saying nothing while listening to those dreadful clichés about "Heaven's Special Child," or "Little Gift from God," or "Angel Sent from Above" just for us? The idea that Ben is a gift from heaven is totally offensive to us. Worse, it is demeaning to our son. Ben is not a cute little kid any more, nor unaware of things said about him. He is a young adult functioning pretty well in the real world. And that's exactly what he wants to be, no more, no less.

It seems to us that if our children who happen to have been born with an extra chromosome are to be considered *fully human* with rights to education, jobs, independent living . . . all those things many of us have struggled and continue to struggle for . . . then we can no longer allow them to be classified as "angels," or "gifts," or "messengers" sent to make us better people, build strength of character, test our faith, show us what love is all about, whatever. *Think about it!* Has the supernatural really intervened and sacrificed the intellect of our children so that the rest of us may benefit in some oblique way? Not *our* kid He hasn't!

But that is just what these dreadful sentiments imply.

Sometimes we find that we have to put our politeness on hold. When people repeat that old line about God knowing what he was doing in purposefully choosing us—or any parents—we ask them outright whether we are to conclude that God is a lousy judge of character when parents can't cope, *no matter what*, and *reject* their child with disabilities.

We've come to the conclusion that if we are to be true and effective advocates for our son, we have a *duty* to tell it like it is. How can we, his parents, expect society to accept him in a realistic way—to respect him as a person, flawed perhaps, but a person nevertheless—if we insist on adorning him with a mantle of the supernatural?

Realistic acceptance is what we all should be striving for. Sentimental glop is not going to do it for our kids. In fact, we're convinced that it promotes the continuation of negative and outdated images.

Alas, there is another extreme which is doing no great service to those with Down syndrome. Some parents are so hung up with "Image" that they read and project qualities into their kids that are not there. They even become angry at those who do not also see those qualities. "My son is a regular teenager." "My daughter is totally mainstreamed in sixth grade (well, except maybe for math, reading, science, and grammar), but she is *totally* mainstreamed." "My kid is no different from any kid on the block." Sorry, I don't buy it. Except in rare instances, most people with Down syndrome are not going to achieve on the same level as their normal peers. This is in no way saying they are lesser. It's honestly admitting that they are different in some ways. More naive? Baffled by third-grade math? Or second or first? Awkward at running and throwing a football and baseball? Stymied by a job application or driver's license test? Limited in career choices?

It's a rare parent who doesn't like to brag at some time or other about his or her offspring. But warning bells really go off in my head when I hear about the kid with Down syndrome who's "achieving everything at a normal level." I've known many, many children with Down syndrome through the years. I've yet to meet one who's made it through a *regular academic* high school curriculum or graduated from college. This is not to say I haven't known youngsters who have done very well, even excelled in certain areas. Ben has a friend whose knowledge of old horror movies—names, places, dates—is phenomenal. He talks so intelligently on the subject he could easily be a guest on a TV talk show.

And although I've never heard of anyone with Down syndrome making it to Major League Baseball or the NFL, Ben does have another friend who is a gifted athlete. Slim and well coordinated, he's a superstar of Special Olympics, but is also involved in regular sports and more than holds his own.

Ben himself is no slouch when it comes to Beatles trivia. His expertise on every album they ever made rivals that of a disc jockey. And he's up on other groups as well.

But this does not mean that these truly engaging young people are on a par with their normal peers at all or even at most levels. If Ben's going to make it, he will have to be accepted for exactly who and what he is—not an *image* of what we, his parents, might have wanted him to be. We cannot as a realistic option "read" things into him that are not there, no matter how we may ache to do so.

If *we* cannot see our children as they really are, how can we expect to be able to straighten out others' perceptions of them? As society increasingly acknowledges that our sons and daughters with mental retardation have contributions to make and abilities to be used, this is something that we who love them *must* be willing to do. We must unshackle them from those kinds of images which, no matter how loving the intent, distort our perceptions of them and their condition.

Some years after Ben's first trip to camp, I came across that old snapshot. There Ben stood, the little boy who is no more. (He *was* cute!) What could I have been thinking to send him off to camp that way? Dressed for a display case, not a rugged hike through the woods. I'd been image making rather than equipping him to function.

In the snapshot he doesn't look retarded at all.

# If

....

O ne morning I was just about to run the dishwasher when the phone in the kitchen rang. It was Ben calling from the public phone in front of the supermarket where he works as a courtesy clerk. "Hi, Ben, how're you doing?" "Fine." "How's the job going?" "Fine." "I'll see you for lunch pretty soon—be careful walking home through the woods." "OK." Click—end of conversation.

I'm not sure why Ben calls me from work almost every day. I suspect he likes dropping the coins in the slots and hearing them clink. Whatever the reason, I'm glad he phones. I enjoy our funny, sparse conversations, if you can call them that. And because knowing how to use a public phone is essential for him, the calls are good practice.

When I hung up the receiver I was still smiling. I stood for a minute looking out the kitchen window. Our backyard—which, even on its best days, could never be a candidate for *Better Homes and Gardens*— was at its mid-winter scruffiest: bare trees, withered tomato vines, no grass (except for onion grass, of course). I've looked out at this scene countless times. We've lived in this house more than twenty years, since before Ben was born. What it was that so jolted my memory on this particular day, I don't know. But suddenly, with painful clarity, I remembered standing exactly where I stood now, looking out the same window at our yard in winter, holding the receiver to our phone, a dial phone then, black, on the wall exactly where our present phone, ivory, hangs.

It was my mother on the phone that long-ago day. She'd called to see how the baby and I were doing. Ben was barely a month old. Allen and I had known for two weeks that Ben had Down syndrome—or *Mongolism*, as it was called in those days. We had told a few close friends the truth about Ben. We had not told my parents, who were three thousand miles away in California, and we had not told Allen's widowed mother, who lived in Allentown, Pennsylvania. There were several reasons for our silence. One, we were still in a state of shock and were trying to deal with the situation day by day, muddling through somehow. Two, we instinctively felt it would be better not to tell them by phone, especially when we knew so little ourselves and were so bewildered and distraught. Three, and most important in this decision, my parents were both in poor health and I did not want them worrying about us, grieving for us. I actually feared that my father might have a heart attack. (He had a bad heart.) Yet oh yet, how I wanted their support—I needed so to have their arms around me even from thousands of miles away.

We had told my parents only that there was a slight problem with the baby—in fact, what *we* had first been told, that the baby had poor muscle tone. True enough. As my mother talked, asking about me, Allen, the other children, and the baby, I felt my resolve weakening. I could just blurt it out and maybe the burden would lessen a bit. I had three—no four—children now, but at this moment of such sorrow and fear I was my Mom and Dad's little girl, and they knew how to make things right. I almost had the words out—we were talking about Ben's muscles—and then I heard my mother say, "Honey, try not to worry too much. It could be worse—it could be *mental*."

There wasn't any question she was talking about mental retardation, and right then I could have said it—Mom, it *is* mental, mental retardation, that's what it is, Mom!—but I couldn't. I could not say those words to my mother, not then, maybe not ever. I can remember holding onto the phone receiver so tightly my knuckles turned white. And I can remember trying to keep my voice sounding normal as tears flowed uncontrollably and I was desperate for a Kleenex. When we hung up, I stood with my head against the wall, hand still on the phone, sobbing my heart out.

But I had done the right thing. There's never been a doubt about that.

If there are regrets, it's in the circumstances that made concealing Ben's condition necessary. The sad irony which has haunted me through the years is that my parents would have been crazy for Ben, and he for them. On our previous trips to California and their trips back to see us, our other kids were entranced by them. My parents were warm and loving but what made them irresistible was that they knew how to play with kids. My father was still one himself, intrigued with magic tricks, yo-yos, jumping teeth, you name it. As a youngster, he'd been in vaudeville and he could sing and dance and play the piano and accordion. He and the late Danny Kaye were cut from the same piece of cloth, and kids just naturally gravitated to him. No wonder ours thought he was the world's best Grandpa. And my mother, tender-hearted and generous; a sad face—human or animal—would get her every time. I firmly believe she still holds the world record for rescuing the most stray dogs and cats.

Her reference to retardation that day was not for lack of compassion. She was trying to cheer me up, to comfort me. How could she know that her words uttered with love and concern wounded me so?

In retrospect, I realized that those words were a reflection of the time she grew up in. Mental retardation was so misunderstood, so entangled with erroneous ideas, and to many the absolutely worst possible thing that could happen to a family. It never crossed my mother's mind, I am sure, that any problem the baby had was other than physical.

Sometime in the future, we would make another trip to California and they would learn the truth about Ben. By then we would know more ourselves and could handle it better, we hoped. For now, not a word.

With Allen's mother we did the opposite. When she came from Pennsylvania, we told her right off. *Seeing Ben in person*, being with him, minimized the impact of the diagnosis. Her calm acceptance was a relief and Baby Ben loved being held and cuddled by her. Even now, though, after all these years, we have never really been sure if she understood the significance of what we told her. She too was of the era when Mongoloid—Mongoloid Idiot—was the prevalent term. But it was impossible to pin such a label on this baby who grew livelier and cuter by the day. Maybe she thought the doctors were wrong. Or maybe she understood that a *baby* is a *baby* is a *baby*. . . . Let the future take care of itself. She was never to see the mature Ben, for she died before he was two.

Meanwhile, Ben was achieving many milestones, almost at a normal rate. But we didn't get to share them with my parents, and it hurt. How could we say, "Ben's sitting up alone at eight months!" Why shouldn't he be sitting at eight months? my parents would have wondered. Why, in fact, shouldn't he be sitting at six months? "Ben's babbling and pre-verbalizing!" Why shouldn't he be? "Ben's crawling lickety-split after the cat!" So what? Don't all babies do that if given the chance? It hurt not being able to tell *the truth*.

You know the old saw about If We Had It To Do All Over Again. Well, we'd do it all over again the same way, given the same circumstances. This is not to say it was an easy decision to live with. It often was the source of deep sadness and a kind of bitter irony.

We had always taken a lot of pictures of the children to send to the grandparents. We still did, only now we censored them. In some pictures at certain angles Ben's face looked flat under his eyes, in others perfectly normal—and very cute. I sent only the "normal" pictures. There was one I still remember: tiny, tow-headed Ben is sitting under a tree with Friskie, the neighbors' dog. My mother wrote back that she and my Dad loved the picture, that Ben looked so much like my brother—long-grown—had looked at that age. "He's just adorable; we can't wait to see him!"

Our loving deception was working.

How long it might have gone on we were never to know. Ben was over a year now and we were tentatively planning when we would go to California and how we would break the news (whether by letter or in person). But we never made that trip. My parents died, both of them, within months of each other. They died believing that all of their grandchildren were healthy and normal.

I repeat, if our particular circumstances were the same (my parents' poor health and the geographical distance), we'd act in the same way. But I believe that the kind of information dearth that partly governed our actions is now gone. Things have changed in twenty years, and are still changing. Not that grandparents might not be ill and live far away. Rather, grandparents and all the rest of us no longer have reason (or excuse) to be victimized by myths based on superstition, error, and lack of knowledge. There is too much good information around these days: books, magazines, newspapers, movies, TV. You would have to live in a vacuum to avoid having at least *some* accurate information. Most important, people with mental retardation are no longer invisible. They are increasingly becoming active members of society.

*Whether or not* Ben had ever been born, if my parents were alive today they would already know something about Down syndrome. If my parents were alive today, chances are they would have met someone who is retarded—in their neighborhood, on a bus, maybe working at the grocery store (it's a sure bet my mother would have stopped to talk). If my parents were alive today they would be free of those images and prejudices which doomed children from birth to lives as useless "retards."

I'd be free, too. Of course, breaking the news that something was wrong with our baby would still be a wrenching task, made more painful by the fact that I was telling the baby's grandparents and I was afraid for them. But eventually I'd be able to say, "Mom, Dad, the baby has Down syndrome. I sure need you."

A few days before his twenty-third birthday, Ben called me again from work. "Don't forget the party things!" "I won't." "The popcorn." "I won't." "The pizza!" "I won't." "The drinks!" "I won't." "OK." Click.

Ben's birthday bash seems to get bigger every year—family, friends, bedlam! A true celebration, a time of joy. How my Mom and Dad would have loved it!

*You know what you think of your child, but what does he think of himself?*
*Believe it or not, I didn't ask  let alone answer—this important question*
*until Ben was ten. The resulting revelation inspired this essay, first published*
*in the Washington Star on August 13, 1977.*

# Ben on Ben

· · · · · · · · · · · · · · · · · · · · · · ·

Something kind of great happened at our house not so long ago.
It was one of those ordinary incidents that in retrospect turns
out to be profound.

We'd had a visitor, a young cousin from California whom we'd not
seen since she was a child. There was true cousinly rapport all around
and most especially with our ten-year-old, Ben, who had not even been
born at the last family get-together.

It might have been the second or third day of the visit—I don't
remember. And I don't remember the conversation leading up to it but
Ben said something funny or unusual, for Cousin Sue shook her head
and with laughter and affection cried, "Oh Ben, you are such a doll!"

Ben stopped in his tracks, gave her one of his looks reserved for
people who are really out of it, and emphatically declared, "I'm not a
doll. I'm a person!"

Now this wouldn't strike a lot of people as remarkable or even make
the "Cute Kiddies Sayings" of the local paper. And although it struck
me as kind of funny when I first heard it I really didn't give it much
thought until hours later when I was falling asleep.

Then, in sleepy reflection, I realized that, indeed, it was a terrific
statement, a very revealing statement and deserving of much more than
passing attention. Ben didn't know it, but his words bespoke the
heartbeat of a family.

The more I thought about what he said, the more jubilant I felt.
The irony of it was truly delicious. Not a bitter irony at all, but a certain
irony nevertheless.

Since Ben was born those ten years ago and we were finally able to accept the irrevocable fact that our beautiful baby would forever march to a different drummer, we have been his staunchest advocates, all of us, mother, father, brother, sisters.

To us Ben has always been a person, loved and nurtured, with no limits set on what he might achieve. In this we are no different from other families with handicapped children. The National Association for Retarded Citizens—one of the best advocacy groups in the United States—was founded, after all, by parents determined to see that society cast off its medieval attitudes toward the mentally retarded and did right by them.

But in all this time of making sure that other people, including ourselves, "understood" about Ben, we never really stopped to think what Ben thought about Ben.

Oh sure, it's always been obvious that he's had a good feeling about himself. Anyone as cocky and determined as he is can hardly be classified as a shrinking violet or in need of ego boosting. Somehow in some way I guess we've been doing the right thing.

But we never really thought to check things out from his point of view, to see life through his eyes rather than always through our own. We've been so busy fighting the world on his behalf, of being advocates for him, that we never stopped to realize that he makes a pretty darned good advocate for himself.

Ben's statement of his personhood shows pretty clearly that our desire to make his life full and eliminate the roadblocks will have to give way to his right to stumble now and again and pull himself up—just like our other children.

I've thought a lot about Ben's words and the positive way that he uttered them. I'm so proud of him that I tremble to think how far he's come.

In those first months after he was born, I used to wonder with apprehension if he'd be able to do things that other kids could do, if he would be aware of the world around him, if he would savor life.

Today Ben is leggy and freckled, a great pizza and hamburger aficionado, and in many ways he's like any ten-year-old boy. But not in every way.

He is what they called moderately retarded. There are those who are a lot more capable than he is and others who are much more severely or profoundly affected. I guess you could say he's somewhere in the middle. And that's his reality, and ours.

Ah Ben. You took your cousin's term of endearment so literally, but that is your way. No, you are not a doll.

And you're not some kind of "cute pet" to be loved but yoked any more than you are some "special little messenger" sent by the supernatural so that we may "all be better people," or whatever. You are none of those things and we who love you do not demean the essence of your humanity by considering you as such.

You are exactly what you said you are, and I like to think you were speaking not only for yourself but for all like you—

"I am a person!"

# Eye of the Beholder

. . . . . . . . . . . . . . . . . . . . . . . . . . . . . . . . . . . . . . .

Sometimes I wonder what people *really* think about Ben. When we are somewhere in public and someone obviously—or not so obviously—looks at him, what is that person *really* thinking?

Better *you* than me . . . He's kind of nice looking, what a pity . . . . I'd rather die than have a kid like that . . . It's great to see him enjoying himself and acting so normal . . . Retards like him shouldn't be seen in public; it's too disturbing . . . How do those parents stand it? . . . He seems like a good kid; I wonder how it happened? —

There are people who meet your eyes forthrightly and you read their understanding and *know* that they too have a relative, or have loved someone, who has a handicap. Others meet your eyes tentatively, wanting to reach out to you but not quite knowing how. Some people just stare, ignorance and downright stupidity written on their faces. (By far the hardest for me to deal with. I have such an urge to berate them, if not punch them out.) Then there are those who turn away because—as instinct tells me—seeing Ben has rekindled painful memories, perhaps of a child who died or was long ago "sent away."

How different it is when one parent meets up with another parent of a child with Down syndrome! There is true communion of spirit among parents of children with Down syndrome; we all know that as a fact of life. There seems almost to be a built-in radar. When we see another child with Down syndrome, we look around for the parents and 99 percent of the time we find that "recognition," like spotting an old friend. Rarely—although I've seen it happen—does the other parent turn away. Most times it's like a reunion, instant rapport, mutual reminiscences.

But most people we chance to meet know little or nothing about Down syndrome, and haven't had any reason to learn about it. We can't be sure what goes on in the heads of those who encounter our kids. Strangers anywhere and everywhere: the shopping center, Joe's Pizza Parlor, the Ice Capades, the next block. Whether our child with

Down syndrome is yet a cute little four-year-old or a young adult, he or she is still going to be looked at, inspected as it were, by strangers. And as often as not, I'm convinced, this "inspection" will be from a prejudged, prejudiced, biased—call it what you will—point of view.

You can have a nondisabled kid blocking the aisle of any grocery store, rolling around the floor screaming for a lifetime supply of ice cream and candy, and, of course, people will stare. But they don't stare in the same way as they stare at a child with mental retardation, no matter how circumspect the child's behavior may be. And if—oh spare us please—ours is the one rolling on the floor, it wouldn't be because the kid might just happen to be a brat. Oh no, this behavior would be because the kid has mental retardation.

What can we do about people who stare? Probably not much. What can we do about the prejudice or ignorance that makes them fault mental retardation for every one of our children's actions? Should we embark on a personal crusade to enlighten society?

When I see someone looking at Ben I try to catch that person's eye. If I see a glimmer of a smile, I smile back. If I see even a hint of hostility or disapproval, I put my arm around Ben and stare back. (Actually, I probably glower.) If someone looks and turns away, I really don't do anything—I haven't figured that one out yet.

Overall, most people look at Ben with kindness, and when they get to know him, with affection. For those who don't, I'm the first to say—Better *me* than you!

# Underestimating?

· · · · · · · · · · · · · · · · · · · · · · · · · · · · · · · ·

**M**any years ago, gifted author Katherine Anne Porter wrote a grim yet poignant short story entitled "HE." It centers on a poor farm family whose youngest son has mental retardation. The parents in this story never give their son a name; he is always referred to as HE or HIM. There is no outright cruelty toward the boy; the father and particularly the mother love him in their own way. But they are bewildered by him, bewildered by the fact that he was born to them at all. They do not exactly view their son as a sentient being. "They didn't talk before HIM much, but they never knew just how much HE understood."

Of course, this is fiction set in another era, the 1920s or a few years before. You wouldn't think something like this could happen in real life and modern times, would you? I wouldn't either if it weren't for a family I was acquainted with a few years back.

This family always referred to their daughter with Down syndrome as "Baby," or "The Little One." Nobody could doubt the love and devotion these parents had for their daughter, but I used to wonder if they weren't doing her irreparable harm. The young lady was almost thirty years old! They would talk about her in her presence as if she weren't there or couldn't possibly understand what they were saying. And maybe she couldn't. She was certainly what would be termed low functioning—unusually low functioning for someone with Down syndrome. She had little speech and could barely do anything for herself. Her parents had not enrolled her in school until she was nine or ten and then only reluctantly. It was very hard for them to let "their baby" go.

Most of us would find what these parents did unacceptable and disturbing. We are distressed by them, even as we well understand the feelings, their desire to protect her, which motivated them. The attitude this mother and father expressed in such loving terms seems a throwback to that other era—and almost surely is. Today's parents—

us—are determined that our children "grow up" and become part of society. In order to make sure this happens, we cannot and do not treat them as perpetual "dear little ones." We make it a point, in fact, to let it be known that in every way possible we are raising our children with mental retardation in the same way we are raising our other children. This has become our dogma—we could write an anthem to this end and maybe we should. But before we do, perhaps we should take a hard look at those parents who saw their adult-age daughter ever as a "little one," *and* at ourselves. It is easy enough to dismiss them as hopelessly out of date. Yet, are we so different from them after all?

Not so long ago, I was talking with another parent about what happens when a child with mental retardation gets upset. This father said that when his seven-year-old son gets mad or sad, the family generally ignores him. "Sometimes he is so cute being mad that we can't stop ourselves from laughing. Does this mean we don't respect his feelings or credit him with having genuine human emotions? Is it because we think him incapable of understanding an explanation that might make him feel better?"

This discussion got me thinking about our attitude toward Ben's emotional needs. Allen and I most definitely do not call Ben "Baby." And the idea of him as a "little one" is pretty ridiculous. Ben's bigger than I am and probably as strong as Allen, who's no Mr. Chicken. But we do wonder if we aren't sometimes guilty of underestimating Ben's *awareness*. Like many people with mental retardation, particularly people with Down syndrome, Ben is not always too skillful at articulating his thoughts and feelings. Therefore, do we tend to downplay those feelings in a way that we do not do with our other children? I am not saying that we do—and we certainly wouldn't do it on purpose—but I fear that sometimes we might, *without even realizing it*. For example, when our girls were teenagers I often used to comment—with a sigh—that raising a son with Down syndrome was a piece of cake compared to raising two teenage daughters. And I *meant* it! Why did I feel this way? Was it because the girls seemed to be forever involved in a crisis of the week? Was it because the events in Ben's life were easier to control and, thus, to deal with by comparison? Or was it that his emotional needs, whatever they might be, did not seem to me to be quite so important as those of the girls?

I remember agonizing when Ann was trying out for the pom-pom dance team in high school. Ann was very shy as a teenager, so this was a major effort on her part and took a lot of courage. I was as thrilled as she was when she made it. A couple of years later, I "suffered" again when Claire tried out for the cheerleading squad, and was again relieved and happy when she too was accepted. But whether or not the girls were chosen for their respective teams was out of my hands. I could encourage them and stand by them, but I couldn't make it happen for them. Nor could I make sure that a boy one of them might have a crush on returned the feeling. I couldn't patch up a quarrel they might have with a friend, and I couldn't make speech class any easier, or less required, despite the many times I heard, "I absolutely can't stand up in front of that *terrible class* and talk!"

If Ben had a problem when he was younger, it just seemed less complicated to handle. If someone teased him in the classroom or on the school bus, I called the teacher to talk about it and the problem was usually solved, or at least addressed, within a day or two. If Ben became upset about something at home or if a trip to the ice cream store did not materialize, we could generally pacify or distract him, promise him a future trip. It worked most of the time and there was no emotional go-round involved, no big deal. Try telling a teenage girl who wants to be a cheerleader that it's no big deal!

There is something else to be considered, though. It is quite possible that during this period Ben's mental retardation did not totally account for the differences in the way we responded to his needs and to those of his siblings. Perhaps we were merely dealing with him as most families do with the *youngest* child whose brothers and sisters are more than a few years older.

There is another type of underestimating that we as parents need to be alert to. That is the assumption that many or most things our child with mental retardation hears us talking about are over his head. When a child is very young, parents can talk freely about that child, and anything else, in the child's presence. (Sooner or later, parents usually have to resort to the old trick of spellings things out, until, of course, the child becomes a better speller than the parents.) Eventually, if parents want peace in the family, they no longer talk in front of the child unless they have a specific reason for doing so.

But when a child has mental retardation, it is so very easy to go on as always. The pace is slower, awareness comes slower, "growing up" is a long way off; we still have lots of time before "the little one" will catch on to what we're saying, don't we?

And some will never catch on at all. Right?

As Ben has gotten older he has continued to amaze us and remind us, too, just how much he *has* "caught on." We do at times underestimate him, not greatly, but it does happen. Once during the war with Iraq, he and I were watching footage of a battle. I saw Ben shake his head and heard him whisper, "This has got to stop." I had no idea that he was so attuned to the news and felt so deeply about the violence of war.

Now that he is a young adult, all of us in the family make every effort not to discuss Ben in his presence, unless it's to praise him or remark on something interesting or significant that's happened to him. He usually dismisses such comments with a shrug or a groan. He doesn't like to be talked about and he doesn't like to talk about himself. We did not even find out that he had received a commendation at work for returning a lost wallet to its owner until the manager saw us shopping in the store and told us. Ben had not said a word.

If that's the way he wants it, that's the way it's going to be. We'll honor his wishes not to make him the subject of conversation, and avoid topics that might possibly wound him. After all, we may never know just how much Ben understands, but it's probably more than we think.

# Unexpected Dividends

. . . . . . . . . . . . . . . . . . . . . . . . . . . . . . . . . . . . . . . . . . . . . .

The last thing I want to be taken for is Little Mary Sunshine's older, dumber sister. Silver linings are OK, but people who consistently sing their praises—with or without music—annoy me. I often have trouble finding silver linings in the first place, let alone singing about them. I freely admit that there are times when I think having a child with Down syndrome is *not* the best thing since Swiss cheese.

Now, having confessed to these pessimistic leanings, I nevertheless unequivocally state that there are some unexpected dividends in being the parent of a child with Down syndrome—tangible and intangible assets that are there for the taking. Those of us who have been parents for a long time, or even a short time, know this to be true. It's almost redundant to say so.

When feeling contemplative, I sometimes consider how Ben has influenced our lives in ways we never foresaw at the time of his birth. How *could* we foresee? At first, when you're so wrapped up in the newness, the unknown, the heartache, you're not thinking about matters like insights and increased patience. You just want to make it through another night. You're not thinking of siblings in terms of finely tuned sensitivity and compassion. More likely you're just hoping they won't be put down because they have a brother or sister with mental retardation. You are not thinking of fulfillment and maturity of spirit for yourself, for your family, for anybody. You're just wishing the whole thing hadn't happened. You have a changeling baby instead of the baby you were waiting for, and lectures about assets and dividends sound like so much twaddle.

Twaddle or no, the dividends do exist and they do influence our lives. I've mentioned insight, patience, sensitivity, and compassion. I could also include the mantle of activism/advocacy which seems to fall on many, if not most of us, sooner or later. Some find a true calling in advocacy, a blossoming of purpose and accomplishment. Others of us just sort of go along for the ride, but at least we go.

Then, who would have thought that we'd end up so knowledgeable about genetics, medical research, special education? True, if we'd had our "druthers" we'd have preferred to read about such subjects at the library (and not have reason to read about them at all). Like it or not, we've learned a lot, and more importantly, we know how to use what we've learned to help our kids, and in helping them, ourselves.

Wait, there's more. Through the years I've talked with many new parents. In giving them information, I always try to be as forthright as possible, positive yet realistic. Often I'm asked if we are glad or sorry that we had Ben, or more precisely, if we would rather have him the way he is than not have him at all. I tell them that we have no regrets about having Ben. There's no dilemma about that. Our dilemma would be if the Happy Elf, Good Fairy, or the like would magically appear and grant us the option of having Ben be normal, not retarded, no Down syndrome. It's when I say I'm not sure what we would do—we might not act on such an option—that I get that look, "Is *she* for *real?!*" I always hasten to explain that for Ben's sake, his own sake, of course we would choose for him to be normal. But for our sakes, his mother's and father's, I'm not so sure we would change him at all.

There are times when Ben's idiosyncrasies, quirky behaviors—call them what you will—drive us crazy! We would be less than honest not to admit it. But there are qualities in Ben we cannot long resist. We find him endearing, refreshing, and innately good. We don't believe for a minute that his "purpose in life" (thanks to an extra chromosome) was to benefit us, but that's what, indeed, has happened. In the end he has done right by us, this funny, beloved son of ours.

Whether directly or indirectly, Ben has been a conduit for bringing some very remarkable people into our lives, people we would never have met under other circumstances. Don't misunderstand me and think "Oh, There She Goes Again!" I am *not* saying it sure is a lucky break for us that Ben was born with Down syndrome because now we get to meet all these great people! But the fact is, certain paths would not have crossed if we had not had Ben, and Ben had not had Down syndrome.

Some individuals have touched our lives fleetingly; others came to stay. There have been doctors such as Dr. Mary Coleman, who has devoted much of her life to research on Down syndrome. Her interest in children like Ben and her dedication to making their lives better inspired hundreds of parents with hope for the future, and that surely included Allen and me! And Dr. Margaret Snow, our family doctor, who looked me in the eye—all weepy and scared as I was—and said, "You treat this baby as you would any baby! He may be a little slow, but he *will* progress. You've had three other babies—do for him what you did for them and he'll come along fine." This down-to-earth advice turned out to be true, of course. Dr. Snow was actually a part of our lives before Ben was born, had been our doctor from the time Douglas was an infant. But she was such an anchor for us during the turmoil following Ben's birth that I cannot think of that period without thinking of her.

There have been nurses, psychologists, therapists, teachers (some super, caring teachers). Each year when we attend the fair at Stephen Knolls School (where Ben went to school before he was mainstreamed), I am touched by all who remember him. His primary grade teacher who taught him to read—and has taught many since—always greets him with affection. The principal, now retired, the speech therapist who used Ben as a role model for fellow students, others of his teachers. "Hey Ben, how are you doing? How's your job? We're so proud of you!"

Then there were the teachers who were involved with mainstreaming Ben and his classmates. How they pushed those kids to succeed and constantly looked for ways to expand opportunities for them! Where would Ben have been without these people—all of them—in his life? And where would we have been?

The prime dividend, though, was meeting those other parents who in the course of time turned into cherished friends, as close as family, maybe closer. I think all of us who have been involved with a parent group have reaped this dividend. I'm not being sentimental here; at least I don't think I am. As with any other group or organization, bonding between members is not a requisite. We're not going to have simpatico with everyone; just because parents have a child with Down syndrome doesn't automatically make them candidates for "Nicest Human Beings to Walk the Earth" Award. As we know full well, Down syndrome is not discriminatory. Anyone can have a baby with Down syndrome, even jerks (and you know who you are).

But what about those who do come into our lives to stay? Those with whom we've shared so much? We came together through fate, and then by choice, our lives entwined forever. It's way beyond Down syndrome now. We've rejoiced with each other at weddings and births, wept and cheered at graduations, worried over illnesses, and mourned deaths. We've bolstered each other, scolded each other, laughed and cried with each other. We've pulled each other through time and again.

What we're talking about is friendship, steadfast and abiding. To me such friendship is a dividend, a by-product of having Ben; value of inestimable worth which no portfolio can match.

Oops, am I sounding like Little Mary here? So be it.

*Since this essay was first published in 1983, I've added considerably to my store of "humor nuggets." These are still some of my all-time favorites, though.*

# He'll Never Sing at the Met

. . . . . . . . . . . . . . . . . . . . . . . . . . . . . . . . . . . . . . . . . . . . . . . . . .

What's a mother to do when her kid stands up in an Italian barbershop and at the top of his lungs—and dreadfully off key—sings out, "Figaro! Figaro!"?

When this happened on a recent much-needed trip for a haircut, I didn't know whether to stare transfixed at the ceiling, deny all kinship and claim the quiet child in the corner as my own, or express the triumph I felt that Ben could equate grand opera with a happening in his own life.

My frantic misgivings about any possible ethnic misunderstanding and my pride in Ben's perception left me in frozen confusion. This was melted almost instantly, thank goodness, by the cheers and applause of barbers and patrons alike as Ben climbed exuberantly into the barber chair.

Enzo, who has cut Ben's hair for years, beamed, "Hey, did you hear that? Ben knows 'The Barber of Seville!' How about that!"

How about that, indeed!

What we have here is what I like to think of as a "humor nugget," a prize of rare worth which I tend to store up to offset those times when there is absolutely nothing funny about raising a mentally retarded child. And make no mistake, there are plenty of those times.

On balance, though, I think I've garnered more "nuggets" than tears. And certainly each member of the family has gained an expanded, if not oblique, point of view. You do not find, for example, too many mothers, fathers, brothers, and sisters jumping up and down for joy because the baby of the family lost his tiny temper and with clarity to please Professor Higgins, uttered, "Damn it! Damn it! Damn it!"

Thirteen years ago when each new word Ben added to his vocabulary meant so much, we didn't stop to think that a "no-no" might be appropriate. It was only hours later that such a thought crossed my mind. I discarded it. As Walter Cronkite used to say, sort of, "that's the way it is" when you have a child whose learning abilities you try to enhance at every opportunity. In my book, it's a lot more uplifting to hear a two-year-old Ben say "Damn it!" than not to hear him say anything at all.

Blue noses who don't agree with this philosophy will be pleased to know that Ben at fifteen is no paragon of virtue. Like other kids his age, he is predictably unpredictable: messy, moody, too noisy, too quiet, stubborn, silly, serious, etc. Not so deep down he is tenderhearted and loving. Popular vernacular would be correct in classifying him as a "typical teenager" in many ways, except, of course, he is mentally retarded.

All of this he is. And there is no getting away from it; often he is terribly funny.

It is downright refreshing to be with Ben and his peers, especially at those times when "the world is too much with us." Today's realities don't often inspire one to stand up and cheer, but there is an undeniable sense of revival in knowing someone who can make a mundane trip to the barbershop a cause for celebration. Seen through Ben's eyes, new dimensions have a way of popping up. American history may even take on unique aspects as we discovered when we toured Jefferson's Monticello a few years ago.

We prepared Ben in a general way, telling him it was the home of Thomas Jefferson, who long ago had been president of the United States. We explained we would be seeing things which had belonged to Jefferson and his family and, yes, we would probably see a picture of President Jefferson himself there at his own house. Ben grasped this easily enough. He likes history, has learned much in school, has visited the White House, and it's easy to see he's a true patriot.

The tour went well with Ben the model tourist until he spied upon the parlor wall a painting depicting the head of John the Baptist being presented to an eager Salome. An anguished "Oh-oh, Thomas Jefferson!" and Ben literally fell to the floor in great consternation, stopping the tour guide's spiel cold. We pulled him to his feet and quickly backtracked to another room, attempting to assure him that it was only a picture and had really nothing to do with Thomas Jefferson.

Too bad for true history buffs; Ben wasn't buying. His unwavering version of that period in America's history is that the unfortunate Mr. Jefferson was done in by "a real mean lady" who put him on a big tray and served him up for Sunday brunch.

There is no doubt that Ben is a literalist, very much from the school of "what you see is what you get." It is part of his appeal and it is surely part of the reason he triggers funny situations.

Ben, for example, will tell you that when somebody sets out to drive a car, he should drive as carefully as possible and avoid crashes. Good drivers don't bump into people on purpose. As he puts it, "That's wrong!" And fie on us that we didn't keep this in mind when we let him solo in a "bump car" at the beach boardwalk a couple of summers ago.

Ben's sense of outrage was stretched to the limit when those "crazy drivers" kept bumping into him and each other with such wild abandon. His indignant shouts could not be heard above the din, but there was no ignoring his furious gesticulations. The other kids didn't understand this at all, but it was not the time for character analysis of a spoil sport.

His dad and I could only hope he would not jump out and attempt to leave by foot. No need to worry. Instead, he managed to turn his little car around and go scooting off in the opposite direction, a fine move until the rest of the pack met him at the far curve, where all converged in one great multiple crash.

When I uncovered my eyes, Ben was the center of a massive traffic jam where all cars had come to a standstill. The man in charge turned off the switch and the ride was over, to the disgust of all the kids, except Ben, of course.

Ah well, everybody's out of step but my Willie.

Now I realize there are those who can't see any humor associated with mental retardation. It's my feeling that this is probably because they are too sensitized to see the person—they see only the condition.

There is no denying that when parents are told their baby has Down syndrome, the sense of anguish and heartbreak is overwhelming.

But the fact is that along life's way sooner or later almost every family raising a Ben will have its own collection of "humor nuggets," a collection which becomes a cherished part of the family tapestry. How can your laugh muscles not twitch when you tell your darling he's the cat's pajamas and he looks at you as if you've just spilled soup at the White House and informs you that "cats don't wear pajamas, you dumb-dumb?"

Not polite maybe; funny surely.

And how limited we would be if we did not accept this gift of life's funny prism. How much narrower our perceptions of what truly is important and what is not.

From La Scala to the Met, partisans of Placido and Luciano vie for title of world's greatest tenor. Alas for them, it will never be settled. For me it's easy. My vote—and my heart—belong to the kid who sang "Figaro" at the local barbershop.

# Still a Rose

. . . . . . . . . . . . . . . . . . . . .

"**S**ticks and stones may break my bones but words will never hurt me!" That old saying is not true, of course, and nobody knows it better than those of us who have kids with handicaps. Most of us can probably remember more than one time that a word directed at our child caused us almost unbearable pain and anguish.

When Ben was a couple of months old, I took him to be examined and evaluated at a clinic then doing research on Down syndrome. It happened that the day we went, a group from a mental health organization was visiting the clinic to learn more about Down syndrome. I was asked to undress Ben and then hand him over to the examining physician, who checked him out thoroughly as he explained what was going on to the visiting health professionals. I sat on a chair at the side of the room watching.

The physician carefully positioned his hand under Ben's small belly and lifted him from the examining table. Ben's arms and legs dangled down and I heard the words, "Here you see the typical *Mongol* with the problem of hypotonia. Notice the lack of firm muscle tone in the arms, legs, and neck, and notice the tonguing. Most *Mongoloids* exhibit these characteristics, which are often the first clues in the diagnosis of *Mongolism*."

As I sat there hearing these words, I was holding Ben's diaper and the spiffy little baby clothes I had chosen so carefully for this visit. Next to me were his diaper bag packed with more diapers, more clothes, his favorite rattle, and a couple of bottles. These were items a loving mother had brought along for her *baby*, her *child*, her *son*.

To this day I cannot hear the words *Mongol*, *Mongoloid*, or *Mongolism* without a vivid recall of the pain and despair I felt on that long-ago day when I watched my unique and precious baby being viewed as a specimen. I am among those who rejoiced when those terms began to be replaced by *Down's syndrome*. In all honesty, though, I don't believe *Mongolism* and its derivatives were deliberately intended to be pejorative. *Mongolism* had been in use for so long that most people didn't think about it, except parents like me, of course, who winced inwardly whenever we heard it.

Why was *Mongoloid* used in the first place and how did the word come to take on such a negative connotation?

It was erroneously believed that the slanted or "oriental" eyes (epicanthic fold) of people with Down syndrome connected them to the people of Mongolia, who are a major racial stock native to Asia. Not surprisingly, these Asian people protested the use of terminology such as *Mongoloid* or *Mongol* to describe people with mental retardation. Their protests stirred the medical community (and parents too) into finding a new and more appropriate name for the anomaly. Eventually, *Down's syndrome* was chosen in honor of Dr. J. Langdon Down, the London physician who originally differentiated these patients from those with other types of mental retardation. (Years later the name was changed to *Down syndrome*, dropping the possessive form.)

But old habits die hard. Check out the medical books and dictionaries and you will find that even in the mid-seventies *Mongolism* was still being used more often than *Down's syndrome* or *Down syndrome*. And the term as ever conjured up a dreadful image. It surely must be because in earlier days the words *Mongoloid* or *Mongolian* were often followed by the word *idiot*. Children like ours were called "Mongolian Idiots." Sometimes "idiot" was dropped after "Mongoloid," but the negative connotation remained.

There are other words which hurt, too. All of us have heard them. *Imbecile*, *moron*, *feeble-minded*, *teched*, and the one which really drives me up the wall and is heard too often, *retard*, used as a noun. Once in a while I have encountered a seemingly intelligent person who says that word in conversation without hesitation and without realizing the utter lack of sensitivity such usage shows. I can't understand this. I would think that anyone with half the sensitivity of a red brick would know the word is offensive when used in such a context. Teenagers who want to insult their friends know it, make no mistake.

When Ben was about nine years old, we were spending some time at our usual summer haunt, our community swimming pool. I was lazing in the sun watching a group of teenagers horseplaying in the water. They were really enjoying themselves—those healthy young kids, splashing and ducking, laughing all the while. Perhaps something happened that I didn't catch, but one of the boys suddenly swam to the side and pulled himself from the pool. He stood there looking at the still frolicking group and then twice yelled very loudly, "Hey, you *retards*—you *retards!*" And then he walked away.

It shot through me again—the pain, the anguish, the fierce anger. I should have been used to it by then, but I never was, and I'm not now. I can never seem to get it through my head that such brutal insensitivity is so much a part of our culture that a savvy teenager uses it quite handily as the gross insult, the ultimate putdown. My first reaction that day was to make sure that Ben, who was swimming nearby, had not heard. Fortunately, this was the case, for thanks to previous instruction by a couple of bratty little boys, Ben had found out that *retard* is a word which makes you hang your head and try not to cry.

My second impulse was to jump up and go hit the young man with my beach towel and give him a lecture. Of course that's all he would have needed in order to become truly enlightened! I didn't do that, but today I think I would, even if the kid considered me to be a batty old lady ranting and raving about a word that's not even a legitimate curse word.

Perhaps other words push the emotional buttons for you as these particular words do for me. No doubt there are words you can barely tolerate, words you'd like to get rid of forever!

Now, having admitted that as the parent of a child with disabilities, there are certain words and terms that bother me a lot, I would also like to point out that there are other words, phrases, and terms that hardly bother me at all. But they do seem to bother some. There are people in the disability field, and a few parents too, who are very doctrinaire about language. To a certain extent, I can understand why. These people feel that if you say, "children with disabilities," you are implying that disabilities are something the children *have*, not something they *are*. You are emphasizing that the children are people first, rather than *disabled* people first. They have similar objections to the use of words such as *handicapped* or *crippled*. You should not say "handicapped child," "disabled person," or "Down syndrome kid." At the urging of these word watchers, the federal government has even gone so far as to rename the Education for All Handicapped Children Act the "Individuals with Disabilities Education Act."

While I can understand the rationale behind these proposed language changes, I fear that such distinctions can lead to cumbersome technology and euphemisms which seem sort of like a denial of reality. What happens when we are talking about our kids with other parents? How many of us, in casual conversation with one another, remember to say "our children *with* Down syndrome" rather than "our Down's kids"? How often do we use the phrase "my disabled child" rather than "my child with a disability"? Do we always remember not to say "handicapped"? If we are in earnest, heartfelt conversation with those we know well, don't we often use the spontaneous, short-cut vernacular?

And, when we go the long way around in order to avoid saying something, doesn't the very avoidance often point it up all the more?

Ben is not a Mongol, an imbecile, a retard. He is not dim-witted, teched, or feeble-minded. But in certain areas he is *not able* to function adequately. In certain areas, he *is* disabled (as in disabled in his ability to do math).

Is there some magical phraseology that corrects the disability or creates instant acceptance of the child with a disability? When we look at Ben, we see *Ben*. When we think about or talk about Ben, it is *Ben* who is in our thoughts. Whether or not we call him Ben who has a disability or Ben who is disabled, our circumstances are the same. Our preference in terminology, one way or the other, has not changed anything about him whatsoever. He is still *Ben!*

A lot of time and effort can be spent in trying to bring language into line as some perceive it should be. And maybe those who feel strongly about it should continue to battle for less casual terminology. Perhaps down the road it truly will serve handicapped individuals—individuals with handicaps—if terminology becomes more precise, more structured. If I may make an observation though, I think energies spent on the critical need for education and job-training programs would be more useful.

It's my hunch that those who take on a "language crusade" will have their work cut out for them. They won't have a great, emotion-rousing banner to carry because words like *disabled* or *handicapped* don't really have the kind of awful baggage attached to them that *Mongolian Idiot* does. The difference between saying "disabled person" and "person with a disability" simply does not have a great degree of emotional impact. (And in fact, the distinction may well be lost on most people unless someone explains to them in detail exactly what that distinction is: a person first, not the disability first, etc., etc.) It does not make me wince if someone calls Ben disabled, a Down's kid, or mentally retarded (instead of a person *with* mental retardation). Frankly, I just can't get that worked up about it, and I suspect that most parents and people in general feel the same way. I see nothing pejorative in those words. They do not conjure up the awful pictures that *Mongoloid, moron, retard, imbecile,* and so forth do; those graphic, visual images of hopeless and useless lives which some of us have imprinted on our memories forever.

Long ago I heard my baby called a Mongol. It wounded me deeply and I grieved that someone could look at him and label him so. Weren't they able to see that above all else he was a baby, my sweet Baby Ben?

Today I would never allow anyone to call him a Mongol. No way! Sometimes, though (and he'd have a fit if he knew), I look at him and I still see my sweet Baby Ben.

# Mainstreaming . . .
# Yes? No? Maybe?

· · · · · · · · · · · · · · · · · · · · · · · · · · · · · ·

Shakespeare's Hamlet might have anguished over "To be or not to be?" but I don't think he was in any more turmoil than parents who are anguishing over "To mainstream or not to mainstream?" To be honest, I'm glad that *that* part of decision making is behind us. Mainstreaming today is more complicated than it was even a few short years ago when Ben was in school.

I believe part of the difficulty lies in the number of ways *mainstreaming* is defined. From what I've observed, the words mainstreaming or integration seem to have a different meaning to different people.

Does mainstreaming mean that a child with mental retardation is put into a *regular* classroom and does the *very same lessons* the other students do?

Does mainstreaming mean that a child with mental retardation is put into a regular classroom and does only *some* of the lessons the other students do?

Does mainstreaming mean that a child with mental retardation is put into a regular classroom with a backup system: a full-time aide to help the classroom teacher, an itinerant special education teacher to provide special help when necessary, a speech therapist, a physical therapist, etc., etc.?

Does mainstreaming mean that a group of children with mental retardation are housed in a regular school but have their own special ed teacher and their own special ed curriculum, and only join the regular student body for physical education, music classes, recess, assemblies, and the like?

If a child is going to school in any of these circumstances, it seems that he or she is considered to be mainstreamed.

How do parents choose the best option for their own child? There are those—special educators, advocates, parents themselves—who push for "total mainstreaming." They believe that being in a classroom with "normal" children of their own age is best for children with special needs. And there are parents who spend a large part of their waking hours making sure that their kids have this kind of school experience. These parents have to know all there is to know about Public Law 94–142 (The Education for All Handicapped Children Act of 1975, renamed the Individuals with Disabilities Education Act in 1990) and be ready to prove to school authorities that mainstreaming can work. They may literally have to build a case as a lawyer builds a case. If a school district is resistant to the idea, parents have to press for the backup team—teacher's aide, therapists, and so on. And that's only the beginning. Once that child is in school, there must be constant communication between parent and classroom and backup team. Is all this effort worth it? Many parents think that it is. They can, in fact, become very emotional about the issue. They are prone to refer to mainstreaming as "integration" or "full inclusion," as if to imply that this is something—like Mom or Apple Pie—that no one could be against.

There are other parents, though, who believe just as strongly that mainstreaming does *not* work, at least where *their* child is concerned. They concede that their child's social skills might improve and that nonhandicapped students may certainly gain insight and under-standing by having a classmate with mental retardation. But as one father points out, his seven-year-old son doesn't really care who his classmates are. "He is very happy and works equally hard whether he is with normal kids or special-needs kids. I'm not fighting some great civil rights cause for mainstreaming; I'm just after the most effective education for my son." The parents of this child removed him from a mainstreamed setting and enrolled him in a non-integrated placement because they thought he was not getting a good enough education. There was not enough backup support at the regular school and the school district would promise no more. These parents felt that their son needed intensive instruction in order to learn, and that he would not get it in a regular classroom. According to them, "Children with mental retardation need well-designed, quality special education to learn; if we expect our kids to read and write, they have to be taught long and hard. Sitting them in a regular classroom is not some magical way of teaching reading, writing, and arithmetic. It is a way of making grown-ups feel good about themselves."

This family's experience points up a major problem. What happens if a school district cannot or will not, for whatever reason, provide the backup to make integration into a regular classroom work *educationally?* Many school systems hard pressed for funds are simply not going to make such provisions. What happens then?

Other very valid questions are raised here. If the child does not care who his classmates are, who benefits from mainstreaming? Does having your child with Down syndrome in a regular school and in *some* regular classes make *you*, the parent, feel good . . . proud? You can say, "My kid goes to a regular school!" But suppose your child is happy in a segregated classroom and possibly better off educationally? In whose interest are you then making the decision to mainstream? And are you shortchanging him?

From time to time, we've been asked whether Ben was mainstreamed in school. The answer is a qualified "yes." Ben was never *totally* mainstreamed, at least by our definition. When Ben and his classmates moved from Stephen Knolls, a school for students with moderate retardation, to Kensington Elementary, a regular school, they went with their own special ed teacher and into their own self-contained classroom. They *did* have a lot of interaction with the rest of the student body because this school had a sensitive and enthusiastic principal who was well prepared to receive them. Another important factor was the age of the students at this school. Kids of elementary school age are for the most part willing to befriend kids who are a little "different." Junior and senior high school students are not always so receptive, can be pretty cruel in fact, although there are always exceptions. Today, of course, there is a lot of emphasis on mainstreaming in the early grades when young children have a great capacity for accepting one another.

The great hope is that this acceptance will carry over into areas of life long after school days are bygone. One of the first meetings on mainstreaming that Allen and I attended, in fact, emphasized this concept. It is not only the people with handicaps who will benefit, we were told, but the non-disabled as well. "Normal" kids who are in school every day with kids who are not "normal" will, hopefully, grow into adults who do not stare or make snide remarks or fear those who are "different."

Looking back, we consider ourselves fortunate that Ben had the opportunity to be mainstreamed as much as he was. Overall, he and his classmates benefited from the experience, particularly the work-study program in high school. (We credit Ben's success on his job at least in part to the program.) But remember, Ben and his friends were not mainstreamed in the early years. They learned to read and write in a school for students with mental retardation. And in that school they were taught well. In addition, they had certain perks such as weekly swimming and bowling which the students at regular schools did not.

Would they have been better off academically if they had been mainstreamed in the first grade instead of what was the equivalent of fourth or fifth grade? Or if they had been placed in a regular classroom instead of a self-contained one? I don't think there is any way of knowing.

I can tell you that every parent of Ben's classmates would opt to do it again. There have been no regrets. But there were certain realities to be faced. Being involved in this program meant long bus rides for some students. It was a real hassle those days when the bus broke down or for some reason didn't show up for the morning pickup, which happened more than a few times!

In high school, there was a new set of realities to face. Here Ben and his classmates were pretty much a hidden population. Their classroom was downstairs in a corridor where other classrooms seemed mostly unused. In fact, I doubt that the majority of the student body even knew these kids were in the school unless they happened to pass them in the hallways. The high school experience of these mainstreamed students was nothing like "Corky's" of TV fame. I'm not being critical; this was simply the way it was.

However, things are looking up. I have a friend whose son with Down syndrome is now attending the same high school. She tells me that there have been changes. The kids still have their own classroom, but it's in an upstairs hall near the others. There is more interaction with non-handicapped students and the special education kids are enrolled in regular physical education classes. My friend reports that her son has made friends with several of the regular students and that many seem to know him and his classmates. They are no longer "the hidden population."

If Ben were a little kid again and we had the opportunity to mainstream him in the early grades, there's no doubt we would do so. We would give it every chance to succeed. But if we came to the conclusion that it was not working, that Ben was getting shortchanged in his education, we wouldn't hesitate to pull him out and send him back to a non-integrated classroom. Nobody would ever convince me that it is hopeless or not worth the bother to try to teach reading, writing, and math to kids like Ben. Improving social skills and raising public awareness about people with disabilities are just not as important.

Mainstreaming can enhance the lives of many children, both with and without disabilities. But I don't think it is set in concrete that it will always benefit every individual. Parents should not be made to feel that they are somehow "traitors to the cause" if they decide that mainstreaming is not in the best interests of their child.

Not so many years ago the question concerning kids like ours was "To educate or not to educate?" and the answer was mostly "No!" Today it is a different question, light years away from the old: "To mainstream or not to mainstream?"

No matter how we answer, I think we can all rejoice that the question is being asked.

# The Pie

. . . . . . . . . . . . . . . .

The pie was set at the back of the stove waiting to be dessert. I wish I could say that I had baked it myself, from scratch, but it came from the grocery store. Sweet and juicy apple, not bad for a store-bought pie. I had sampled a piece before returning it to its box and setting it on the stove.

Ben and Laura—twelve years old at this time—were due home from school any minute. Later they'd be going to Special Olympics. Each Tuesday we alternated with Laura's parents; one week Ben would go home on the school bus with Laura and eat dinner at her house, after which her folks would drive them to Special Olympics and then bring them home. Today it was our turn.

Sure enough, in they came. They greeted me, dropped their gear, headed for the kitchen to fix snacks and then down to the rec. room to watch TV.

All was peaceful, but there is something you should know. If ever a youngster belies those "experts" who advise that children with Down syndrome are passive and lack imagination, it is Laura. Irrepressible, headstrong, savvy, compassionate Laura; with Laura one is wise to expect the unexpected.

I was upstairs changing into sneakers (a good idea as it turned out) when I thought I heard the front door open, then close. I wasn't sure. But there was no mistaking the terrible squawk I heard from Ben! When I ran downstairs I found him pulling open the door. "Laura's run away with the pie!" And out he bolted. I followed him and he was right! There was Laura fleeing up the sidewalk clutching the pie box close, a regular Eliza. Ben took off in hot pursuit, gesticulating wildly and yelling for Laura to "Bring back that pie!"

As I started to run after them, I saw Laura cut across a neighbor's lawn and disappear between two houses, Ben not far behind. I continued to trot after them but they far outpaced me. Breathless, I slowed to a stop. What was I doing? This was ridiculous. "I'm not going to chase around this whole neighborhood after a damn pie!"

I went home.

Back in the kitchen I set the table for dinner, muttering to myself about what I would like to do to Laura, and trying to figure out a substitute dessert. Part of me wanted to strangle her, the other part chuckled at the image of her running with that pie and the indignant Ben so desperate to catch her.

About twenty minutes passed. I was considering going out again to look for them when the front door opened. In came Ben holding the pie to his chest. "The pie is back!" he announced triumphantly. Laura was right behind him looking as pleased as Ben. Another successful adventure—almost.

Ben carried the pie into the kitchen and sort of leaned over to put it on the table. It must have been an awful angle, for the pie gently, silently, swiftly slid out of the box and landed on the kitchen floor. Triumph to tragedy in one terrible splat! Poor Ben, his look of horror said it all. Even Laura became subdued.

"I tell you what, maybe we can fix it," I said, knowing a repair job was impossible. They both stared at me; they knew it was impossible too. I took a spatula and scraped the pie up and dumped it back in the pie tin. The thing was lumped up in the middle, so I flattened it out as best I could. The kids were watching me all the while. "Do we have to eat it?" they asked.

"I don't know. I don't know what I'm going to do with it. But let's not tell Dad about this."

Did I serve it for dessert that night or not? Remember the famous tale of "The Lady or the Tiger"? It ends with the reader left to guess which of two closed doors the hero chooses to open. Well, I had options too! Keep the pie in the box and pretend I knew nothing about its mangled appearance, mold it into some kind of "dump pie" and serve it hot with ice cream melted on top, give up and throw the mess down the garbage disposal. . . . *You* figure out what I did!

Now, this all happened several years ago. Today Ben and Laura are young adults, out of school and holding jobs. Laura, irrepressible as ever, has found her niche. She works at a nursing home and has a variety of duties. running errands, helping to serve meals, taking residents in wheelchairs for walks. The residents, especially those who rarely have visitors, look forward to having Laura around. I can't be absolutely certain that if given the chance Laura wouldn't make off with another pie. I do know for sure that up at the nursing home she's captured many a heart.

# Their Brother's Keeper?

· · · · · · · · · · · · · · · · · · · · · · · · · · · · · · · · · · · · · ·

Not so long ago, families were often advised, "Don't bring that baby home" because it would be such a "hardship" on the other children. A young woman I know reports that her parents were told exactly that. Thankfully, the old myth has been all but laid to rest now. These days, the overwhelming consensus seems to be that having a brother or sister with Down syndrome enhances siblings' lives in many ways.

Most adult siblings I know profess to having deep and meaningful relationships with their brothers and sisters with mental retardation. Many avow that it is the most special relationship in their lives. I've often heard them say things like: "Tim is my closest friend. He has more love to give than anyone else I have ever met. He is sensitive to my feelings and really knows if I am feeling down, upset, angry, or sad, when no one else does. He always tries to fix whatever is wrong—even if it is beyond his control."

Besides growing to love their brothers and sisters for themselves, siblings often grow in other ways, too. Most grown siblings agree that because of their brother or sister, they are much more empathetic to anyone with a disability. They feel they have gained more compassion and understanding than they would have otherwise, and consider this gain a definite plus. And many learn the art of being patient, which often does not come easy, especially for teenagers. I think of Douglas, ten years older than Ben, who would let Ben come into his room to listen to records. Pesky little brothers are not always allowed in such a sanctuary, but Douglas put up with him and, in fact, first introduced Ben to the Beatles. Doug had no way of knowing at the time that he was providing Ben with one of the truly great joys of his life. He had simply become aware that Ben had an ear for music, so he played records for him. Douglas is not by nature particularly patient, but with Ben he managed to be, and both benefited from it.

But don't forget: en route to developing these loving, mature relationships, most "normal" children have to make some hefty trade-offs. Having a brother or sister with retardation is not always a picnic, nor does it always make for a more beautiful life. Often siblings have to cope with feelings and concerns that can be a darn heavy load. Nobility of spirit has its limitations, especially when smothered in platitudes. I'm afraid that sometimes, probably more often than we know, our "normal" kids suffer in silence while putting up a good front for us.

Often our children's worries and concerns are born along with their brother or sister who has mental retardation. Ann, for example, has recently confessed that she had moments of near despair at the time Ben was born. Ben spent the first month of his life in the hospital, not because he was sick, but because he was part of a research program conducted at the old Children's Hospital in Washington, D.C. We had explained to our children that the baby would be coming home in a few weeks and that he was *not* sick; they were just running tests on him. Evidently, eight-year-old Ann didn't buy this. She convinced herself that her baby brother was going to die, and she had never even gotten to see him! She kept these terrible fears to herself. She would cry at school, but refused to tell the teacher why she was upset. She cried herself to sleep at night, quietly into her pillow so we wouldn't hear her. To "spare" us, I guess, she never said a word about it, and at that time we were so concerned with Ben that I know, in retrospect, we did not give her the attention she needed and deserved. Until the day Ben came home from the hospital and she saw him for the first time, Ann suffered greatly. And we never knew.

Even when siblings are more than a few years older than the new baby, the wrenching shock of their brother's or sister's birth can leave them reeling. One young woman who was a teenager when her sister was born confesses to deeply resenting her mother's pregnancy in the first place. "It didn't seem right." When the baby was born and turned out to have Down syndrome, it compounded her resentment because her parents were so preoccupied with the baby. "All they thought about was the baby!" Eventually love, aided greatly by maturity, won out, but for a long time this family was in turmoil with a very unhappy sibling.

Another sibling who was about fifteen when his sister with Down syndrome was born also went through a lengthy adjustment period. His parents were obviously very upset about something having to do with the new baby, but they offered him no explanations. This disturbed him greatly. Why wouldn't they talk to him about it? Later, after the diagnosis was confirmed, his parents were quite forthright with him and said that they had been too uncertain about the baby's condition to try to explain anything to him. Even so, years later, he still feels they should have included him from the beginning no matter how worried and confused they were. He didn't see his parents' silence as "being spared"; he viewed it as being "left out." As much as he loves his little sister, the time period of her birth still brings back painful memories.

Parents' concerns do not cease at the end of the neonatal period, and neither, of course, do siblings' concerns. But when we are caught up in our own worries, it is all too easy to overlook signs of our children's emotional struggles. Ben's sister, spunky little Claire, usually stood her ground with everyone and seemed to let things roll off her back. But she was so deeply anguished about an incident that happened when she was in fourth grade that she couldn't bear to tell me. I only found out about it many years later when we were discussing how having Ben as a brother had affected her childhood. Claire remembers vividly that some boys in her class were throwing the word *retarded* around in a derogatory and insulting manner until she could stand it no longer. It hurt so much, she said, for Ben and for herself, that she jumped up and shouted for them to stop it, that her brother was retarded. The boys laughed at her. "Ha, ha, I guess it runs in the family!" Claire was stricken to the heart. Those boys made her feel so ashamed and mortified that for many years she avoided telling anyone that she had a brother with Down syndrome.

Years later in high school, Claire became close friends with a classmate named Susan. The first day Susan visited our house and met Ben she said, "Why didn't you tell me you had a brother with Down syndrome? Do you know that another friend of mine has a brother with

it? They're neat kids! It's no big deal—why didn't you say something?"
On that day, a burden was lifted from Claire and she realized the
difference between a mature point of view and the ignorance of childish
insults. (Susan, by the way, grew up to obtain a master's degree in
sociology and now works with people who have severe handicaps.)

All three of our now-grown children have told me something about
their childhoods which should be of particular interest to parents who
are activists and doers. Back in the days when I was very active in our
parent group, I was frequently on the phone with new parents—sometimes near desperate parents—and I also wrote numerous letters and
articles and devoted a lot of time to advocacy. It was my way of "doing
something," and I *needed* this outlet. I guess it was a form of therapy.
My children have admitted that at the time, they didn't understand
*why* I was so *busy*, and *why* I didn't hang up the phone when they
wanted me to stop and talk with *them* instead of someone else. *Why*
was I so preoccupied with other people and *why* did it always seem to
have something to do with Ben? Ann, Claire, and Doug too have
confessed to feeling a certain resentment and to deliberately misbehav-
ing, especially when I was on the phone, in order to get my attention.
(Have you ever tried to sound calm and upbeat on the phone while
you're trying to catch and smack your kids at the same time?) *Now* they
understand what we were dealing with, but at the time they did not
and they faulted me for "neglecting" them.

Do I feel guilty about this "neglect"? In all honesty, I do not. I could
say I wish I had done this or I wish I had done that, but without benefit
of hindsight I would probably do the same thing. With that hindsight
in place, however, today I *would* cut back on my activities *and* I would
encourage my children to tell me what they are thinking. I'd like to
believe that I'd say something like: "Don't be afraid to hurt our feelings
or think you are going to upset us. It's very important that we be honest
with one another. If there is a problem, how can we make it right if we
don't know what it is?"

As children approach adulthood, move out of the house, and put
some space between themselves and their brother or sister, they often
gain a new perspective on family life. At times, it may seem as if they

can look at everything quite objectively. For example, many siblings think their parents are too easy on the child with Down syndrome, especially if that "child" is now an adult. They generally opt for stricter discipline and for parents to "follow through." "Mom, if you say he can't go out to shoot baskets until he puts his shoes away—then stick to it!" Our three children have told us more than once that we are not tough enough on Ben, although they concede that being tough is a full-time job and can be exhausting. Like many other siblings who think their brothers and sisters are somewhat spoiled, Doug, Ann, and Claire think the same about Ben. (I always say, "Look who's talking!" when they indulge him in french fries and Slurpees.) But it's true. We spoiled him and probably still do.

Another opinion adult siblings often share is that parents are too slow to grant independence to their brother or sister. But some of them concede that parents have no real guide as to when to let a child with mental retardation go off into the world. Most kids reach age levels when certain events are expected to take place. You go to school dances, you go on a date, you take public transportation alone. But what age is a kid to do these things when the chronological age is not the same as the mental age? As one grown sister says, "My brother is so innocent, so vulnerable. My mother wants to protect him. I think that is good, but it can be frustrating for him when he knows he can do something and nobody will let him."

A dilemma we all know too well.

Although adult siblings may appear detached at times, make no mistake, they are still emotionally involved with their brother or sister. If nothing else, they are bound to worry about what the future will be like when their parents are no longer around to care for their sibling with mental retardation. Ann in particular has given the future a lot of thought. She's asked me whether I think that sometimes—maybe often—siblings mouth sweet platitudes (He's the best thing to happen in our family—there must be a reason—she's so loving—they're such joyful children, etc., etc.) because it is easier than admitting some of the true feelings which can take over now and again. Feelings like resentment, anger, sorrow, unwanted responsibility (it's your kid, *you* had him, I didn't). How do you come to terms in deciding what you owe to yourself in your own life and what you owe to your brother or sister?

Ann tells me that this last question is always in the back of her mind.

Obviously, Ann and Ben are very close. At least once a week, usually more often, Ann comes by to do something with Ben: to go out to lunch, to buy a soft drink (he treats), to go shoe shopping, or to take him and one of his friends to a movie. Ann is very generous in giving her time to Ben, but this generosity has created a worry for her. She is concerned that if she should marry and have a family of her own she won't have as much time to spend with Ben as she does now. She fears he would be hurt and not understand. What if she had to leave the area? What would happen to him?

We have told Ann again and again that she cannot and must not put her life on hold in order to cater to Ben. We have pointed out that sooner or later Ben will go to a group home and that Ben not only has a job, but a pretty full social life, thanks to his many friends and the activities he shares with them.

But even though Ann was once a counselor in a group home and thinks Ben will do very well in one, she still worries. Suppose the group home turns out to be unbearable? unacceptable? It can happen, she says, due to turnover in staff, poor management, whatever. Or suppose Ben is lax in his grooming and is asked to leave? (We do have to be on his case constantly.) Or suppose he has other problems?

*And* will people treat him decently in this society?

Ann being Ann will never stop asking these questions. We try to reassure her, as well as Claire and Doug, that we have done everything we can think of to protect Ben (and them) once we are no longer here to watch over him in person. We have consulted the best lawyer we know to write a will so that Ben will be provided for. (Parents have to be very careful about leaving money to their children with handicaps because they could possibly create one *big headache* for their "normal" kids to contend with. If a person with disabilities living in a state-supported facility receives an outright inheritance, the state can make claim to it and use it for highway construction or football stadiums if it wants to.) We have joined a trust association whose purpose is to keep tabs on Ben's interests no matter where he is living or where other family members might be. We have him on lists for group homes and have joined the organizations sponsoring those homes.

In short, we have tried to ensure as bright a future as possible for our children, *all* of our children, in as much as any parents are able to do.

Allen and I need to believe that Ben will be OK without Douglas, Ann, and Claire having to be or to *feel* totally and forever responsible for him. We know that they care, and they will always care, but Ben must be able to lead a life independent of them, aware that their love and concern are there for him, and for each other, sort of like a pot of nourishing soup keeping warm on a back burner, ready whenever it's needed.

Isn't that the way it should be with brothers and sisters?

# When We Walk the Same Mile

. . . . . . . . . . . . . . . . . . . . . . . . . . .

One of the best things that ever happened to me was getting involved with a parent group. It didn't happen right away, though. Ben was nearly two years old when I attended my first meeting. It wasn't only my first meeting, it was the first meeting of our group. It was held at my house and I'm the one who set it up. Even after all these years, I still sometimes find this hard to believe.

I didn't just wake up one morning and think—Hey, I'm going to start a parent group! It was more that I fell into it because circumstances made it the logical thing to do.

When Ben was born we had the opportunity to enroll him in a research project which involved not only an in-depth study of Down syndrome, but also an attempt to ameliorate the physical and mental aspects of the condition. *No promises were made* that there would be noticeable improvement. This was bona fide research funded by federal grants, and involved double blind studies under strict regulations. In this research, some of the children were given daily doses of a substance which researchers believed *might* lessen the physical and mental deficiencies of Down syndrome. Neither the researchers nor the parents knew which children were getting the "real thing" and which were getting the placebo; hence the term "double blind."

At the time of Ben's birth, the clinic doing the study was quartered in the old Children's Hospital in Washington, D.C. For the first months of Ben's life we reported to the clinic every Tuesday; later it was once a month and eventually every few months. But Ben's early life was geared in large part to the clinic and, thus, so was ours.

At first it was a time of despair. How I dreaded Tuesdays! And no wonder. One purpose of the study was to determine whether there was some reason the level of an amine called serotonin is usually lower in people with Down syndrome. So that Ben's serotonin levels could be analyzed, prior to each visit to the clinic I had to collect a twenty-four hour urine sample from Ben using a catheter-like collection bag. The bag was attached to a plastic tube and emptied into a plastic bottle which had to be kept cold. To chill the urine, Allen figured out a system using an ice bucket, a beautiful one surely meant for better things and donated by a loving friend who felt sorry for us and wanted to help. The hard part was keeping the urine absolutely pure; I had to watch Ben like a hawk to make sure a messy diaper wouldn't ruin the perfect sample.

From Monday morning to Tuesday morning, I was sort of like Rapunzel locked in her tower. When Allen came home from work he would spell me, but those hours alone "guarding the urine" were very stressful and I would get awful headaches. I am not very good at doing things with my hands. The prospect of having to manage this procedure, and for twenty-four hours at a time, absolutely threw me. I was in utter turmoil. Why oh why couldn't Ben have just come home from the hospital like any other new baby and be done with it?! Instead we were tied to never-ending medical procedures and endless trips to the hospital. I hated it! But I guess the old adage of "Where there's a will, there's a way," is true. Within a few weeks, I became so adept that I could have made a fortune hiring out as a special nurse. But not at first.

Then something began to happen. Each time we went to the clinic, we saw other parents whose babies also had Down syndrome, some a little older than Ben, some a little younger. And we were all there together, bewildered, scared, hurt, sad, and yet somehow coping, or putting up a good front. We were together in another way too. We were united in hope. It's pretty safe to say that none of us would have agreed to let our babies become part of experimental research if we had not had hope. We weren't even sure what that hope was.

Perhaps a few parents were hoping that their child would be "cured." But I believe most of us were more realistic. Allen and I did not know what it might mean for Ben or his future. But we figured that if something significant were learned from this study, it meant that Ben's life would have meaning for perhaps thousands of children with Down syndrome yet unborn. That thought was a great uplift for us.

Each week we'd see familiar faces along with new faces and their new babies. And we began to talk to one another. Some of us probably would never have given each other the time of day had we met under other circumstances, but now we had a common bond, even if we didn't quite realize it yet. As the weeks went by we all actually looked forward to clinic day. Where we had dreaded it—I had not been the only one to dread it I learned—we now couldn't wait for Tuesdays to come around. We could even exchange funny stories about the urine collections (if people knew the truth about that beautiful ice bucket, they would drink no libations at our house!). Tuesdays became a conduit for a positive charge. We were all putting a lot of effort into our kids, and at the clinic we could share our highs and lows with those who could best understand.

Most of the families who attended the clinic were from Maryland, Virginia, and the District of Columbia. But people came from other parts of the country, too. One time we even met a couple who had flown in with their baby from Rome, Italy. The clinic seemed such a going concern and so much a part of all our lives that we pretty much took it for granted.

Then disaster loomed suddenly. Because of federal cutbacks in a new administration, the clinic was in grave danger of losing its funding and was very likely to close. The research would come to an abrupt halt, a victim of political expediency. Remember that this was a time when Down syndrome was still called "Mongolism" and nobody gave much thought to Mongolism except, of course, those of us who were parents and a few dedicated doctors and teachers. It is safe to say that finding the cause of Down syndrome—Mongolism—and a way to ameliorate its effects were not high on anybody's political agenda.

When I first heard about the clinic's possible demise I was very depressed. Then I got mad! Now, I certainly was no activist. From time to time when I'd felt strongly about something I'd written a letter to the editor and I'd done volunteer work for school-board candidates, but mostly I minded my own business. However, the thought of the clinic closing and its unique and valuable research going down the tubes galvanized me! I sat down at my typewriter and began cranking

out letters to members of Congress—our own senators and repre-
sentatives and others I thought might be helpful. I kept at this for
several days and then that old light bulb went on in my head. Hey—
why am I doing this *alone?* How about all those other parents from the
clinic? Wouldn't they want to do the same thing and wouldn't it be
more effective if those members of Congress received letters from a
whole bunch of us instead of just me?

I called the clinic office, told the doctor what I wanted to do, and
requested the names and phone numbers of the parents who attended
the clinic so I could call them up and get them to write letters. When
the list came to me a few days later I started making phone calls. The
response was terrific! Almost everyone I talked with was eager to join
"the cause."

One of those calls turned out to have far-reaching consequences.
On the list was the name of a mother whose three-year-old son was not
technically a part of the research but had been used as a control. The
children involved in the actual research had to be infants when
admitted to the program and this little fellow was past that age. Even
so, here was a mother vitally interested in keeping the clinic going and
more than ready to do battle on behalf of Down syndrome. Her name
was Celia Wyman and she was later to become one of the founders of
the National Down Syndrome Congress.

Celia lived in Virginia; I lived in Maryland. Many miles and the
Potomac River separated us, so we first came to know each other by
phone, and it was by phone that we planned our strategy to save the
clinic.

First, we had to make those Congressmen we were writing to think
that we were more than a handful of desperate parents. They had to
believe we were an organization with clout! We had to come up with
something that seemed genuine, so right there on the phone we
declared ourselves an organization and decided to call ourselves
"Mothers of Young Mongoloids." If there's one thing to be said about
Celia and me it was that we worked fast! By today's standards our name
choice sounds awful, but remember, *Mongoloid* was the term of the day.

We also decided that to make it seem really official we'd need a letterhead, something that would enhance our badgering efforts. But the letterhead needed names on it, and addresses and phone numbers. I don't remember which of us came up with the idea that Celia would be Area Chairman and I would be President of the Maryland group. We prevailed upon three other mothers, Dolores Baker, Karen Milligan, and Cynthia Siemens, to become Presidents of chapters in Virginia and Washington, D.C. All of our names would go on the letterhead. This was probably akin to stealing an election, except there was no election. But we didn't stop to think about that, and nobody objected. If all this seems to you reminiscent of Lucy and Ethel—or perhaps Laurel and Hardy—you are right. But it worked. To make it even easier, Celia's son-in-law—who was a printer—got us a terrific discount. Everybody pitched in to pay for the letterhead, and we were in business!

In the months that followed, we bombarded Congress with letters, and got our friends and relatives from all parts of the country to do the same. On December 3, 1969, the day when funding for medical research concerning mental retardation was going to be considered by a Congressional finance committee, about fifty of us took our kids to the halls of Congress and lined the corridors outside the meeting room. We hoped that our presence would signify how important this funding was. I still remember how the various senators going in and out of that room looked at us and at our kids, and we looked back. It was an exhilarating experience never to be forgotten. And they voted to fund it!

Certainly in part because of our efforts, the clinic was saved and carried on its work for many years, although it was often faced with financial disaster and threats of closing. More than once it was saved at the last minute.

In the weeks, months, and years to follow, we found we had some very talented parents amongst us. One of these was Paula Felder, who had been a professional fund raiser before her marriage. Her expertise proved invaluable and in time she became a volunteer, almost full time, and an integral part of the clinic's financial management. Federal grants were harder and harder to come by and Paula was forever scrambling to come up with private resources. Somehow she managed—how I don't know.

Ben was a research subject until he was about eleven years old. Our whole family was actually a part of it. One time, blood was needed from "normal" kids for a comparison study. Douglas, Ann, and Claire volunteered to give their blood and so did several of the neighborhood kids. This was no quick blood test either. It involved sitting absolutely still for about fifteen minutes while blood was very slowly taken from the arm and transferred into a special container. The kids hadn't bargained on this and they were all *very apprehensive*, but they did it! They felt they were doing it for Ben.

Much data about Down syndrome was gathered from this research program; as far as I know, some of it is still being studied. The one obvious, *undisputed finding*, though, is that children with Down syndrome benefit in measurable degree if they receive early, constant, and intensive stimulation. The children who were a part of this detailed research all received a great deal of attention from the day they were born. No child was accepted into the program unless the parents were deeply committed to their child and to the aims of the research. The upshot was that almost *all* of the children in the study—those on the substance, those on the placebo—progressed at a faster rate than previously observed children with Down syndrome who were not part of any study. This conclusion was arrived at before early intervention and infant stimulation were much thought about. True, here and there the concept was just getting started. But this study proved that most children with Down syndrome *need* and *greatly benefit* from exactly these kinds of programs—learning experiences beginning on Day One.

In the long run, the most important upshot of our association with the clinic turned out not to be the work done there, but what happened to the parents. Without quite knowing what we were doing, Celia and I had started a Down syndrome parent group. The nucleus at first was composed of parents from the clinic, but it didn't take long for other parents to find us. On both sides of the river, we began holding coffees, informal get-togethers that came to have great meaning for many of us. Sometimes we had speakers, "experts" from various fields, and I always tried to include someone from our local ARC who had abundant information to hand out. Now and then we had joint meetings, picnics, or parties so that all of us from both sides of the river could get together. We also published an "information kit," which became a huge success. We got requests for it from all parts of the country and even from other parts of the world. Celia found someone to translate it into Spanish and we could no longer keep up with the demand. Fortunately, our local ARCs agreed to take over the mailings for us and helped us to pay for revising and updating it several times.

But the coffees were the glue which held us together; little kids crawling about mashing cookies on the floor, someone always ready to hold a baby and make a fuss over it, quiet one-on-one conversations, lively exchanges, questions asked, questions answered, sometimes tears, more often laughter. Informal and seemingly chaotic, they were akin to a spiritual renewal for many.

One mother, now a cherished friend, remembers how she almost didn't come when she first heard about the group. She was afraid it might be too formal, too organized, too proper. She arrived with her two sons, a toddler and her baby with Down syndrome, and the idea that she would leave in five minutes if the meeting turned out to be as stuffy as she feared. We can laugh about it now—the relief she felt when she walked through the door into friendly and welcoming bedlam, and how she was one of the last to leave that day.

The other day, a friend and I were reminiscing about the "old days." We were remembering people who'd been a part of our group, some perhaps briefly; but with lingering impact nevertheless. Ninety-nine percent of our fellow members had children with Down syndrome, but there were also a few parents who had children with other disabilities. There were no parent groups for them to join, so we welcomed them gladly.

One young mother would come carrying her eighteen-month-old daughter. The child, who had beautiful golden curls, would lie in her mother's arms as though asleep—a miniature sleeping beauty. She would remain that way during the whole coffee. She *never* awoke. Another mother would bring her child who had Cri-du-chat (Cry of the Cat) syndrome, a disorder causing severe retardation and an elongated body. Those of us with kids with Down syndrome felt lucky because we knew she had it a lot harder than we did.

I still vividly remember the mother of the small, frail baby with Down syndrome who struggled for every breath. He had a severe heart defect which was apparently inoperable. Today it might well be a different story, but that little fellow wasn't going to make it and we all knew it. So did his mother and she could barely speak without tears flowing. I think we all felt that in some way we were letting her down and we didn't know how to make it better. I don't know if coming to the coffees helped that poor young woman or hurt her. The problem was that the rest of us had high hopes for our children and she had no hope at all. We tried to reach out to her, but what could we say? And what could we do? She only came to a couple of coffees. We heard that the baby had died and we tried to call her, but there was no answer. I wish we could have helped her and I hope that in time she found some measure of peace.

For most of us, though, those coffees helped us face our realities with a certain equanimity. At a time when we were vulnerable, they served us well. We found them to be uplifting, invigorating, and downright fun!

Our coffees lasted for many years. People came and went, but a surprising number of us stayed put. One who left, though, and oh how I hated to see her go, was Celia. She and her husband retired to a small town in Southern Virginia. Celia bequeathed me all that beautiful letterhead, which by then was obsolete, not only because Celia's address was no longer valid, but because the term *Mongoloid* was fast being replaced by *Down syndrome*. I ended up using the letterhead for scratch paper, and we changed the name of the group to "Parents of Down Syndrome Children."

I never did order any more letterhead. None of us in Maryland wanted to be highly organized and we maintained our informal status.

Other changes were coming. Attendance at the coffees began to drop. I think there were three main reasons for this. First, as our kids got older, we of necessity became involved with their schools, with their outside activities, and with myriad projects, and most of us had other children in school as well. Second, as more mothers entered the work force, they were not able to attend morning coffees. (Fathers had never been excluded, by the way, and had shown up from time to time, but we were mostly a mothers' group.) Night meetings didn't fare much better. People were too busy and tired. Third, there were a lot more resources available, and schooling, including preschooling, was now the norm. In our area, there were infant stimulation classes and mothers could meet and get to know each other there. The coffees didn't seem that necessary any more, and so they just sort of faded away.

Today, if someone were to ask me what I honestly thought about joining a parent group, my answer would, of course, be based on my own experience. I would say that I can think of few things more nerve-wracking—for me—than facing a bunch of strangers. The idea of encountering people you do not know at a time when you are vulnerable and in emotional turmoil with fears of the future and countless unanswered questions swirling about in your head may seem overwhelming. More new parents than I can count have expressed such anxieties to me. I tell them, "Look, go to *one* meeting. Bring your husband with you or your mother, a friend, a neighbor. You don't have to stay. Nobody's going to make you join anything, and you don't ever have to go back if you don't want to. But I'll bet you your baby's first tooth that you *will* go back, and will hardly be able to wait until you can!"

I would say too that inexperienced parents can come together and accomplish more than any of them probably ever thought possible. How were we able to start our group in the first place? How were we able to keep a research clinic going? Publish a booklet which became a huge success? Most of us had little or no expertise when we first met. Drawn together by a common problem none of us had asked for, we rose to the challenge. I believe that just about anybody can do the same thing.

Finally, I would say that becoming part of a parent group motivated me toward personal growth and accomplishment and was probably one of the really smart things I ever did for myself. . . .

There *is* a question to be raised. What about families who live in areas of the country—and abroad—where there are no parent groups and little or no resources? Through the years I've received letters and phone calls from many people, and the hardest to respond to are the ones who tell me that where they live there are *no* early intervention groups, *no* preschools, little or *no* support systems of any kind, and *no* other parents to talk with. Where can they get information so they can help their children?

The only really practical step I can tell them to take is to join a national organization, several in fact. Join the National Association for Retarded Citizens, National Down Syndrome Society, National Down Syndrome Congress. The excellent newsletter put out by the Down Syndrome Congress is a lifeline for anyone who can't be part of an in-person group. Imagine feeling isolated and out-of-touch and then receiving a copy of that newsletter and all that it contains! It helps to know that you are not quite so alone after all.

I'm happy to report that Parents of Down Syndrome Children continues today in our area. The Virginia chapter is part of the Down Syndrome Congress and is well organized and going strong with many activities. A Maryland chapter is making a comeback with younger parents of children with Down syndrome. Sparse attendance at morning coffees is still a problem, so an attempt is being made to hold night meetings and include both mothers and fathers, as is done in Virginia. Perhaps "new blood" bringing new enthusiasm will do the trick. Hopefully, when these parents come together to share one of life's really tough handouts, they will discover a source of solace and strength found nowhere else.

I wish them well, for we truly do need one another.

# It's Curtains for the Cat!

· · · · · · · · · · · · · · · · · · · · · · · · · · · · · · · · · · · · · · · · · · · · · · · · ·

A couple of years ago, something sad happened. The cat died. This was not just any cat, this was *our* cat, Diane—or, as we'd called her in her youth—Diane, The Fair. We'd had her for eighteen years, since Ben was a very small boy. Ben had learned to walk by trying to catch the young and frisky Diane. He couldn't even remember a time when she was not part of the family.

Diane was affectionate, sweet-tempered, and not overly flaky, as our other cats have proved to be. In her last two years, though, she developed diabetes. I kept her going by giving her insulin shots twice a day, twelve hours apart as instructed by the vet. Administering the shots was pretty easy. The hard part was crawling around under furniture and poking into corners trying to *find* her. Often Ben helped me; he seemed to know where to look. That old cat had more hiding places! Sometimes I would search for half an hour or more before ferreting her out, not the best way to start the day before that first morning cup of coffee.

Once I found her in the clothes dryer— *after* I had turned it on. When the terrible thumping began, I immediately turned the machine off and flung open the door. To my utter horror, there she was, all limp and goggle-eyed, but no more so than I was to see *her* there. I burst into tears thinking for sure I'd killed her. But within an hour, she was the same old Diane bugging me for food. And that night, she was back to sleeping at the foot of Ben's bed.

When Diane got sick that last time, we took her to the vet as usual. I think we all expected that somehow she'd return to us as she had many times before. But it was not to be.

When the vet's office called to tell us Diane had died, we were all brokenhearted. Ben took the news especially hard. He had a difficult time accepting the idea that she wouldn't be around any more, waiting for him to feed her or pet her, or curled up at his feet each night at bedtime.

We decided to retrieve Diane from the vet and bury her in the backyard. We explained to Ben what we were going to do and that he would be able to "visit" Diane's grave and bring her flowers if he wanted to. This idea seemed to please him.

Ben was in school the morning we brought Diane home and laid her to rest at the top of the yard near the vegetable garden. Like Ben, I could hardly believe she was gone. She had been with us through many a family crisis, and she had given us her total trust and devotion. Once she had even sought us out to deliver a litter of kittens on our bedroom carpet, an event of momentous importance at the time! Our kids, including Ben, were awed and thrilled and never forgot it. (We had Diane spayed shortly thereafter—but oh what fun those kittens were! And we found homes for all of them, except the one that was accidentally swallowed by the boa constrictor at the zoo, but that's another story.)

So many memories of that dear, old cat! I am not ashamed to admit that as Allen shoveled the last of the earth over her I was wiping away a torrent of tears.

Allen went off to work and I glumly busied myself around the house. A couple of hours later, the doorbell rang. It was a delivery man with a huge box containing the living room drapes we had ordered a few weeks before. I signed for them and put the box on a living room chair. The box was very heavy. No sense opening it until Allen was there to help me lift the drapes out and hang them, and they'd probably need ironing anyway. I went upstairs to do some cleaning and forgot all about the delivery.

Around three thirty, Ben arrived home from school. He called, "Hi Mom, I'm home!" And I called back, "Hi Ben, I'm upstairs!"

Silence enveloped the house, which is kind of unusual when Ben's at home. Maybe he was in the kitchen getting a snack. But the silence didn't last long. Ben was coming up the stairs, slowly, ponderously, as if struggling under some heavy load. Even from the bedroom I could hear him huffing and puffing. Then I heard him mutter to himself, "Diane is very heavy!" To say his words jarred me is an understatement, because I knew full well that Allen and I had buried Diane in the backyard that very morning!

I rushed into the hall in time to see Ben stagger into his room and deposit the box of drapes on his bed. "You're back," he said and put his hand lovingly on the box.

You know that old question, "What's a mother to do?"

Well, what *is* a mother to do when her kid thinks that his beloved, late-departed pet has been returned to him neatly packaged? Do you laugh or do you cry?

Ben looked so pleased about Diane's seeming return that I barely had the heart to tell him the truth. I knew I had to, though. Number one, I wasn't about to put off replacing our shabby living room drapes just so Ben could sleep with that box. And number two, I realized that Ben still didn't have a clear understanding of what death was all about.

"Ben, that's not Diane in the box."

"Yes it is. She's going to stay on my bed tonight."

"No Honey, that's not Diane in there."

"Yes it is and she's going to sleep on my bed."

Again I told him no, she was *not* in the box. (And I might have added that even if she had been, I wasn't going to let him go to sleep with a dead cat on his bed!)

He didn't believe me. No amount of talking would convince him that the cat was *not* in the box. Finally, I got a knife and opened up the box and showed him the drapes. Only then, engulfed in sadness, did he accept the truth.

Later that afternoon when Ben felt ready, he went out in the yard with me and I showed him where Diane was buried. We stood quietly for a few minutes and then he wanted to go back into the house to have a snack and watch TV.

Within a few days the drapes were hung and the box was taken away with the trash. Life resumed its normal routine and other cats came and laid claim to our hearts. The little unmarked grave at the top of the yard became overgrown, and Ben didn't go up there much any more.

Sometimes, though, Ben still speaks of Diane. He remembers everything about her—how she liked to eat, how she liked to hide, how she liked sitting outside in the sun, and mostly how she liked sleeping on his bed at night. "I miss her," he'll say. "I still miss her."

That's how it is, Ben, when a good friend goes away.

# Two Hours without Ben: Joy and Fear of Learning to Let Go

. . . . . . . . . . . . . . . . . . . . . . . . . . . . . . . . . . . . . . . . . . . . . . . . . . . .

Somewhere along the line many parents of children with mental retardation face a decision both crucial and frightening. While other parents are chewing their nails over learning permits and college costs, we are agonizing over job sites and bus schedules. Dare we? Should we? Can we?

Can we possibly let our son or daughter go it alone in the outside world?

A year before he was graduated from high school, Ben was given the opportunity to work part time in a hospital cafeteria, getting on-the-job training as a member of the cleanup crew. It was a real chance for Ben to prove himself in an actual community setting.

The plan was that three days a week, Ben would take public transportation from his school to the hospital, and when he finished work he would take a bus to a shopping center where his Dad or I would pick him up. In due time he would be taught how to transfer to a bus that would bring him within walking distance of home.

From the first, Ben loved the job. Aside from lunch (Ben has no use for those who criticize hospital food) his favorite endeavor was removing clean utensils from the huge dishwasher, sorting them, and stashing them in the proper receptacles. But his duties were varied and he learned many skills, basic though they were. More important, he learned to be a job holder.

During the first week on the job, Ben was taught how to take the bus. The job coordinator rode on the bus with Ben and two other students also in job training. When the kids felt comfortable about riding alone, the job coordinator followed them and the bus in his car. Because he can read and knows his numbers it took Ben no time to learn which were "his" buses.

We instigated one rule. Each day when he got to the shopping center, Ben was to call me. I would then know he had gotten that far and should be home within twenty minutes. Admittedly, this phone requirement was more for my benefit than his, but he was more than willing, and if nothing else it gave him added practice at using a public phone.

On the day Ben soloed, he was doing a lot more than returning from work. He was making a journey from the realm of perpetual childhood to his niche, albeit limited, in the adult world. He would not have to be a little boy forever.

It was routine in no time. But on the days he worked, I became a clock watcher until he called from the shopping center to tell me he was about to board the bus. Twenty minutes later, he was home. One day he was about five minutes late. He casually explained that he had missed his stop and had gotten off at the next one and walked back. His self-assurance was contagious; it was time to show our faith in him and relax.

Did we relax too much? It was heavy on our minds as we spent torturous hours one day not knowing where Ben was. He called me as usual from the shopping center to say he was getting on the bus and that was the last we heard from him. He didn't come home.

One hour after Ben's call my husband arrived from work and found me pacing the floor. He turned right around and headed for the shopping center, following the bus route to see if it had broken down. I set about calling parents of the kids who sometimes traveled with Ben (they hadn't been with him that day), the bus dispatcher (no report on him but they took my number), and the police (the police dispatcher would not take his description by phone but said they would send a police officer to the house). Between all the calls my husband was able to get through to say there was no sign of Ben and no broken-down bus.

He returned briefly to check with me and then went back to wait at the shopping center in hopes that if Ben had actually boarded the wrong bus, the driver would help him get back to his starting point.

I couldn't think of anyone else to call and I walked all over the house, upstairs and down, but I avoided Ben's room. I was so scared and so cold, a coldness that went down to my feet.

The phone rang—I hoped that it was Ben—but it was Ben's friend, Craig. I think I told him Ben wasn't home and I hung up and called the bus dispatcher back to check, but there was nothing. I paced around the living room and saw daylight was ebbing fast. Where were the police? I called them again to remind them my son was mentally retarded (I hated using that) and it was growing dark. "They're on the way."

It was an hour and a half since Ben had called. The unthinkable kept creeping in. Had someone spotted him, perhaps talking to me on the phone? Maybe even observed his routine for days and then approached him? The kids were trained not to go with strangers, but how do you train against reality? There is no way to know what they might do in a given situation. We worry with our normal children to be sure. But the added vulnerability of our youngsters with mental retardation also adds to our agony when something goes wrong, because it is our choice to let them go, and, in so doing, we know we are also choosing risk. Talk about a Catch-22.

The phone rang—oh please—but it was Craig again. I think I told him Ben was lost and hung up because I needed to keep a free line.

I went outside and looked down the street. It was very quiet, no one to be seen, and sadness overwhelmed me. If Ben were coming home on his own he would have been here by now.

Ben had been gone more than two hours and it had been one hour since I had first called the bus dispatcher and the police. I called both back emphasizing again that my missing son was mentally retarded. They had nothing new to tell me.

Back in the living room I didn't want to look out the window and see how dark it was and know that Ben was out there somewhere alone with night coming on—or was he? How cold and calm I felt. Maybe this is how it was to die of fright.

Craig called for the third time. I have no idea what I said as I hung up. At least I knew the phone was working. It rang again immediately. Please Craig, Ben's not here, he's lost, gone. Ben is missing!

It wasn't Craig. It was a young man asking if I had a son named Ben. A stranger's voice asking if I had a son named Ben. I went weak and held onto the kitchen table. For a few seconds I couldn't comprehend what he was saying. And as great drama has a tendency to peak at opportune moments, it was right then that the front door opened and in came my husband from his fruitless vigil at the shopping center. The young man on the phone was telling me Ben was OK and that's all I needed to know as I shakily handed the phone to my husband so he could get directions.

As we were walking out the door to go for Ben, the police arrived.

It took us about twenty minutes to find the house, deep within a residential area about six miles from our house. We knocked on the door and when it opened, there was an exhausted Ben standing in the living room. His face lit up with a big, relieved sort of grin and he came and put his arms around his Dad and me. The young man, truly the Good Samaritan, told us he had happened to look out of his living room window and had seen this boy—Ben—trying to flag down cars. A cab stopped, but then sped off leaving Ben crying and visibly upset. So, to our eternal gratitude, the young man went out to see what the problem was and immediately sized up Ben's situation. We have mixed feelings here because this was "a stranger" and Ben went willingly into his house. Ben told him his name and phone number, and the saving call was made.

We have since pieced together "Ben's Big and Awful Adventure" and have concluded that it is not just a matter of one kid getting lost. It goes beyond that. It reaches into the community, and the operative word is awareness.

We know that Ben got on the "right" bus at the shopping center, but for some reason after Ben was aboard, the driver changed the number and destination. The driver does this from inside the bus by turning an overhead crank, and we had warned Ben about it, telling him that if he saw the driver turning that crank he must ask the driver the bus number and where it was going. But Ben almost surely didn't ask, possibly he forgot, maybe he just didn't notice, had gotten complacent. Whatever, he ended up on the wrong bus.

We know that he cried, probably told the driver that the bus was going the wrong way. He made some kind of fuss, there's no doubt of that. It's a sure bet he was noticed. And he was wearing his "Handicapped I.D." bus pass on a chain around his neck. All drivers should recognize that pass.

The driver had him get off the bus.

We know that he walked, several miles at least, and ended up somewhere in a large housing development where each house looked like the other. Apparently, none of the cars he tried to flag down stopped for him except the cab which left him crying in the middle of the street.

Cabs have two-way radios, don't they? Would it have been so difficult to contact the police, through the dispatcher, with a description and location of a distraught, obviously handicapped kid?

Because a decent young man endowed with plain common sense happened to look out his window, Ben spent the night snug and safe in his own bed instead of lost and terrified in the night. Ben knew his name and number; the young man knew what to do about it. Ben got home.

It seems to us this equation could have been used at any point during the time he was missing. But it wasn't, not by those who serve the public; not the bus driver, not the cab driver, not the police who wouldn't take Ben's description by phone while it was still daylight.

The day after our ordeal, I had a very hard time. I wanted like crazy to keep Ben home for the day so I would know where he was every minute. I had a great need to do that. But I didn't. I sent him back, back to school, to the job, to the bus. They had a big discussion in the class about what had happened to Ben.

I think the kids know what to do. It's the rest of us I'm worried about.

# The Cringe Factor

. . . . . . . . . . . . . . . . . . . . . . . . . . . . . . . . . . . . . .

I'd wager that about 95 percent of us have suffered from the "Cringe Factor" at one time or another. You know the scenario. You are talking with someone, almost always someone who doesn't know you very well, a person who has become aware that you are the parent of a "special child." And then you hear it. "You're so *wonderful*—you're certainly doing a *marvelous* thing—it's really *remarkable* how you're handling it—you're an *inspiration!*"

I know that when people spout stuff like this they mean to be kind, understanding, and supportive. But when it is said to me, I absolutely *cringe* inside. I feel as if I'm shrinking up as small as possible—almost as if I've done something perfectly *awful* and am erroneously being praised for it. I often grit my teeth because I am so sorely tempted to reply with sarcasm. "Oh yes, I'm being named Parent of the Century next week—the ceremony will be in the Rose Garden of the White House. The President is going to kneel before me and present me with a certificate proclaiming that I am truly a wonderful person!"

In truth I've never said much of anything when confronted with such goo. "Uh—well—uh—but—gee—uh" is about all I've ever managed to come up with.

What are you *supposed* to say, for crying out loud?

We didn't ask for this, not one of us. For the most part, we all expected to have nice, normal, average (whatever that is) children. We might have harbored not-so-secret longings to produce a genius, possibly a Nobel Prize winner, the future leader of the free world. (And a doctor, lawyer, engineer, teacher, scientist, writer, etc., would do in a pinch.) We had no desire to be "different" from other families.

Most of us can probably think of someone whom *we* would consider to be truly brave, courageous, unselfish, and so forth. I always think of our neighbor and close friend who took care of both her aging parents for years. Her father, disabled by several strokes, managed to get around the house with a walker more or less on his own, but her mother was confined to a wheelchair with Parkinson's disease and was totally helpless—she could not so much as lift a spoon to feed herself. These two infirm people could never be left alone, not even for the duration of a quick trip to the drugstore. Every time she left the house, my neighbor had to arrange for someone to be there. Often it was me, so I became acutely aware of the physical and emotional energy it took for her to care for those poor old folks. It was almost beyond reckoning. I know that *I* could *not* have done it day in and day out, even with a willing spirit.

I was particularly close to the mother, and visited every day. After each visit, I would come home and thank my lucky stars that Ben can do just about anything for himself. It's true that eventually the elderly parents died and my neighbor was freed from her tremendous responsibility. Ben is still our responsibility, but he is also a success story! We do not struggle day by day just to keep him going, all the while watching him deteriorate before our very eyes. Oh no, our neighbor is the remarkable one, not us.

I have figured something out, though. Those who extol us are obviously still influenced by attitudes of a bygone era. They have not yet truly acknowledged that kids like ours can and should find a comfortable niche in mainstream society. As a result, they see *us* as faced with a horrendous problem that, thankfully, is *not theirs*. They want to say something—anything—to make us, and themselves, feel better, so they come up with effusive platitudes. I certainly can't fault people for trying to be kind, but I cringe just the same.

And I really long to say to them—You think Allen and I are so *wonderful*, so *remarkable*, and—the one that always gets to me—so *inspiring*? What *exactly* are we *supposed* to do? How *else* are we to behave? How are we *expected* to function? What *choices* do we have when faced with the fact that our child has Down syndrome?

Do we mope and weep and mourn for the rest of our lives, in the process turning any other children we may have into individuals just as handicapped, albeit in a different way, as our child with Down syndrome? Or do we get on with the business of living, to the fullest possible, for *all* our family members? The choice is just plain common sense to me. And I see nothing *noble, inspiring,* or *wonderful* about it. What I *do* see is survival! Self-interest, when you come right down to it.

No one is saying it's not tough, sometimes very tough. "Might Have Beens" can hurt a lot, especially in the early years. You see neighborhood children riding bikes or playing ball with ease and skill while your little one—who may not be so little any more—has a much harder struggle to master what other kids pick up instinctively.

Those neighborhood kids go off to kindergarten, get promoted to first grade. Yours enters the realm of Special Education. Even if your child enters a regular school, sooner or later the curriculum will be *different*—the road taken will be *different*—the goals will be *different*.

And what about the long haul? That's a question that haunts a lot of us. When Ben was first born, I was terrified at the thought of all the years ahead. How could I possibly last that long? Cope for that long? By nature I am impatient, anxious to get things squared away. I can't *stand* waiting! (As a kid I always did my homework immediately, not out of any virtue; I just wanted to get it over with!) So how would I manage for the long haul in raising a child with mental retardation, especially when I was convinced it would get harder and harder? (It doesn't; it just becomes a series of different ball games.)

Today I find it a significant irony that Ben has turned out to be one of the all-time great Beatles fans. At the time he was an infant, a big hit on the airwaves was the song "Yesterday," certainly one of the most beautiful tunes ever written by the Beatles. It was played all the time and to me became a kind of theme song. "Yesterday, oh yesterday, all my troubles seemed so far away. Now it looks as though they're here to stay. Oh I believe in yesterday." Every time I heard the song, I would think how true those lyrics were, and often I would cry.

But that was long ago!

Allen and I were recently discussing Ben; I forget in what context. Probably we were talking about the one hundred and one pairs of shoes he seems to own and which we're running out of space for. I asked Allen if he ever thought any more about what Ben might have been like if there'd been no Down syndrome. Allen shook his head. "Not really.

Once in a great while maybe, but mostly it never enters my mind. We did what we had to do and Ben is Ben. We've accepted him as he is all these years; why now conjure up an *unknown* Ben who doesn't exist and never did?"

Allen's words probably reflect what most of us who've been around a while feel. What sense is there in looking back? Today we have every reason to be proud of Ben and we are certainly not dismissing all our efforts in raising him by engaging in a ritual of false modesty. We've done a good job with him—a *great* job in fact, and we know it!

And isn't that the point? *All* of us, with mighty few exceptions, have done (and are still doing) a *great* job with our kids! We *have* to. We have no other choice. Either give it our best shot or let our family's well-being go down the tubes. For this we are remarkable? Wonderful? Inspiring?

I don't see it that way. I see it as an act of self-preservation; ordinary parents in a somewhat extraordinary situation doing the best we can for ourselves and those we love most. An honest label: self-preservationist. I can admit to that . . . and I'm not cringing.

# Self-Awareness?
# Self-Acceptance?

· · · · · · · · · · · · · · · · · · · · · · · · · · · · · · · · ·

O ne Sunday morning Ben came into the bedroom to ask me something. There were newspapers spread about, among them a Sunday supplement featuring a story about a group of dancers with mental retardation. A picture accompanied the article. The dancers, both men and women, were wearing flowing garments which looked very much like long, diaphanous gowns. One of the dancers was grinning broadly, and without reading the caption it was hard to tell whether this dancer was a man or a woman. It was obvious the person was "different."

When Ben saw the picture, he got very quiet. Staring at it, he said, "I don't like the way that woman is smiling. I don't like that picture!"

I knew this was a potentially ticklish subject, so I chose my words carefully. "Well Ben, those people in the picture are dancers—that's why they're dressed the way they are. The person smiling is a man. He's very happy because he loves to dance."

Ben didn't say a word; he just kept looking at the picture.

"Do you know something? The dancers in that picture are all handicapped—they are mentally retarded—and they are very good dancers. People buy tickets to see them dance. What do you think of that?"

Whatever he was thinking he wasn't about to tell me. He gave the picture a final glance and left the room.

This episode got me to thinking about Ben's self-awareness. Does he know that he is handicapped, mentally retarded, "different"? Does he have any idea what "handicap" means?

I am sure that he *does* understand the meaning of "handicap," but we have never discussed it with him. The reason we haven't discussed it is because Ben doesn't *want* to! Even when Ben was a young child, he showed no interest in talking about being "different," whether in relation to himself or someone else. We therefore saw no reason to broach the subject with him. For the most part, Ben has always had a strong sense of himself, and, as a psychologist once told us, a highly developed personality. One time, and only one, when Ben was still in school and the class had apparently been talking about handicaps, did Ben say, "I'm handicapped." But he didn't elaborate and has never brought up the subject again.

Ben is not alone in taking this stance. Several of his friends behave the same way. Mara and Paul, for example, absolutely will not discuss the subject of handicaps as it pertains to them personally. Like Ben, they leave the room if the conversation starts to focus on them in any way.

Ben and his friends have certainly seen their share of people with disabilities. They have always had friends and acquaintances—many of whom are mentally retarded—who use wheelchairs, crutches, or braces. Mara, in fact, works in a nursing home. Every day she is with people who are infirm or disabled. Being around people with visible handicaps is routine for all of them.

And yet, I still sometimes wonder how Ben and his friends view *each other*. When they look at one another, do they see any handicap? Do they see that they have a common bond because of a handicap? Or do they simply see a friend with no handicap at all?

And what do they see when they look in a mirror?

Even after many years of being with them, I am not sure if they are aware of a mutual handicap. If they are aware, then it is obvious that it doesn't matter to them. Their friendships are deep and abiding and they accept each other as they are—no judgments, no biases.

I can only conclude—and the other parents agree with me—that these particular young people have come to terms with their state of being. This is not to say that they don't have moments of distress, triggered by a picture in the paper or any number of things. But whatever they may feel about their own handicap, they do not let it get in the way of their day-to-day living. They have never expressed a desire to be anybody other than themselves.

Of course, just because our kids seem to have come to terms with Down syndrome doesn't mean that we don't wonder and worry about how much they know and whether they are suffering inwardly from their own self-image. What can parents do about any anguish their children may be concealing? Allen and I have concluded that if Ben has come to terms with it, so must we. By this I mean that if Ben ever wants to talk about his feelings, his retardation, his limitations, Down syndrome—whatever—we are ready and more than willing to talk with him. The subject is not taboo in our home. Ben has probably heard us talking about mental retardation or Down syndrome in a general way; we do not start whispering or stop talking when he enters a room. But any conversation he might wish to have with us on the subject *he* will have to initiate. We will never make the first overt move. Allen feels, in fact, that to do so would be destructive to Ben's self-image. "Hey Ben, let's talk about mental retardation, Down syndrome, and *you!*" Why should we attempt to start a dialogue when Ben has a healthy ego and a good acceptance of himself, and, as he has made abundantly clear, doesn't *want* to discuss it? Should we *force* him to talk about it? No way!

Parents of children who are much higher or lower functioning than Ben will probably have a different experience. I think, for example, that parents of lower functioning children are spared a certain anguish. In all likelihood, they will never have to worry about how much their children are aware of their own condition and whether that awareness pains them. We cannot say for sure that people who have severe or profound retardation are totally oblivious to their own limitations, but in most cases they probably are. These parents have plenty of problems to contend with, but the problem of their children's awareness is usually not one of them.

Some parents will find themselves in a situation that others might envy. These are the parents whose children *are* aware of their own Down syndrome, who *accept* it, *talk freely* about it, and go on with the business of life. You might be able to think of one or two youngsters you know who are like this, but personally I find that they are the exception (except in the media). At this point, in fact, I'm not acquainted with anyone who has Down syndrome and wants to talk about it.

There is yet another group of parents whose kids also want to talk about Down syndrome, but have a hard time accepting that *they* have it. These are the "Why Can't I?" kids. I think their parents walk a rough path. What do you say when your teenager asks, "Why can't I drive a car?" "Why can't I go to college?" "Why don't the girls in my class want me to go to the mall with them?" "Why can't I go out with the guys on Saturday night and drink beer?"

One of Ben's acquaintances wants to date "normal" girls. He has a hard time understanding why he can't call them up, ask them out, and be accepted just like that. "Why won't they go with me? How come they always say no?"

I also have a friend whose daughter with Down syndrome is actually taking driver education in school and so far is passing the course. She spends hours every night doing the homework required, homework it takes the other students fifteen minutes or at most half an hour to do. This youngster is absolutely determined to drive a car. What a dilemma for her mother! Imagining her daughter out on the streets driving scares her to death. The thought that her daughter might flunk the course or the driving test offers little relief, because if that should happen the girl will be devastated.

Here is someone with Down syndrome who functions at a very high level—close to normal, but *not* normal. She is "mainstreamed" in a regular high school and longs to have friends who are in the "normal" population, to *be* one of them. She reads romance novels and yearns for a romance of her own, with a non-disabled boyfriend. This teenager has told her mother that she thinks people with Down syndrome are "ugly," and she doesn't want "to have it." No wondering for this mother as to whether or not her child is aware. And what can a parent do when a son or daughter out and out says, "I hate Down syndrome! I hate being mentally retarded! Why can't I be like everyone else?"

I have no idea how I would answer such questions and I'm very glad I haven't had to. My friend bolsters her daughter as much as possible and tries to build up her self-esteem. She tells her that not everyone gets accepted just because they want to, and that non-disabled people sometimes have a hard time making friends too. Life can be tough for anyone whether you have a handicap or not. All you can do is be yourself and do your best.

She's right, of course. Life can be tough.

Even nondisabled children sometimes long for friendships and experiences that may never come about. It is an awful anguish for any parent to see their child on the outside looking in. But those of us who have a child with mental retardation may feel more than anguish when we think of other kids rejecting our own. We get angry, resentful, sometimes bitter. Why do others have to be so cruel, or at best, indifferent? Why do they reject our kids? Don't they realize how much they can damage our kids' self-acceptance?

But is it really out and out rejection?

Ben, for example, has acquaintances at work, people who like him a lot. In fact, he considers them to be his friends, and in a way they are. But what interests do they have in common with Ben? What kind of in-depth conversations would they be able to have with Ben about the economy, the state of the world, politics, the best buy in a new car? Would they enjoy hours of hearing him talk about the Beatles, the Three Stooges, high-top boots, what's for lunch and what's for dinner? And how about Ben? At what point would a three- or four-way conversation be over his head?

My friend whose daughter so longs for "normal" friendships in school tells me that this is a major problem; that as sharp as her daughter is, eventually conversations get beyond her and she feels lost, left out, frustrated. Do you fault the other kids for this? Do you say they are *deliberately rejecting* this girl? Are Ben's fellow workers *rejecting* him when he is no longer able to keep up with them, to understand the more subtle nuances of conversation? Keep in mind that these people *do* talk with Ben, exchange pleasantries with him, kid around with him, help him out on the job if he needs it, and even push him to excel. But they do not gear their own abilities to his for those hours he is on the job. This is a workplace in the real world. If Ben loses out on a lot of what goes on around him, that's the way it is. Likewise, when kids at school carry on conversations that are over the head of someone who is "slower," I really don't think this can be classified as rejection. I'm not talking about those who tease or are deliberately malicious to people with mental retardation, the kind of stuff that often goes on in junior high, or which is perpetuated by ignoramuses in general. That is a different issue. I'm speaking about ordinary give and take, the ability to *communicate* and to *share common interests*; two prime ingredients in the making of friendship.

I can't help thinking here about the concept of mainstreaming. There are those who believe that if kids with disabilities are totally mainstreamed, beginning in preschool and continuing through the whole school experience, friendships with fellow students and children in the neighborhood will be almost automatic. Sorry, I don't think this is realistic, or, as the old Gershwin song says, "It Ain't Necessarily So." For all the benefits it brings, mainstreaming is no panacea, as the experiences of the "Why Can't I?" kids clearly show. I am not speaking against mainstreaming. I am merely pointing out that it is not a given that close friendships—or any friendships—will develop between disabled and non-disabled students. Parents can hope that such friendships will come about, but should not be surprised if they don't.

One thing we know, or ought to, is that friendship can't be forced. We can't step in and say, "You *must* be friends with my kid." We can't even say, "*Please* be friends with my kid." As much as we may want to, we can't *make* friendships happen for our kids.

What it boils down to is this. As fervently as we wish for life to be good to our kids, reality dictates that some things are beyond a parent's power to bring about. We just can't ensure happiness for them. We can spend lots of years and lots of effort boosting our child's self-esteem and make it more likely that he or she will grow up to be happy—most of the time. But somewhere along the way, our child will have to make peace with his or her limitations. And this is as true with our "normal" kids as it is with our kids with disabilities. As parents, we too have to accept these limitations in those we love and make our own peace.

Nobody said it would be easy.

# Wanted . . . Fresh Blood!

·················································

When Ben was very young, Allen and I joined our local Association for Retarded Citizens (ARC) and started attending the monthly meetings. It didn't take us long to realize that a certain pattern had been established. At almost every meeting, the same two or three parents would stand up and talk about the dearth of programs for their children, who were children no longer. It didn't matter what the listed agenda might be or whether an invited speaker was present. Sometime before the meeting ended, those parents managed to turn any discussion into a diatribe about problems of adults with mental retardation and their families. Every point those parents made was valid. And I am sure that in standing up and speaking out they were venting deep and heartfelt frustrations. Unfortunately, they were also turning people off. They would monopolize the meetings for many minutes, and I can remember how I kept fidgeting and glancing at the clock. Those of us with small children could barely visualize— and didn't want to—those years ahead and the whole new set of problems they would bring. We were still coming to grips with the knowledge that we had a retarded child—a cute, *little* retarded child. It disturbed us, and, I confess, bored us to hear those "older parents" go on and on.

Today I understand those parents very well . . . their concerns at lack of programs, their worries about their adult-age children who were sitting at home with nothing to do, their fears about what might befall those "children" when their parents were no longer around. There's no doubt those parents were suffering from *burnout*. In retrospect, I think it was amazing and to their credit that they were still attending meetings and speaking out, even if it seemed to others a redundant and futile haranguing.

What about this problem of *burnout?* Let's be honest here. Don't you sometimes get plain tired of thinking about Down syndrome? Of reading about Down syndrome? Of going to meetings about Down syndrome? Not tired of your child, mind you—but oh so tired of the all-consuming subject of Down syndrome?

Wouldn't you sometimes like to forget you've ever heard of chromosomes, flexible joints, speech development, sinuses, Social Security Disability forms, or "Siblings United"? And truthfully, aren't you occasionally turned *off* by those who seem to be perpetually turned *on* by Down syndrome, or more precisely, by Down syndrome as The Great Crusade? I'm talking about the people who seem forever to be going to meetings, symposiums, conferences—who think and talk of nothing but Down syndrome or mental retardation. Don't you long to shout, "Enough already! There are other things in life, for heaven's sake!"?

If you've had these feelings, then welcome to the club. You've got a case of burnout! And from what I've observed, a lot of parents come down with burnout sooner or later, except maybe for the zealots.

The kind of burnout I'm talking about here is, of course, not the same as the kind often suffered by those who must cope year after year with a child with profound retardation and physical handicaps, aged and infirm parents, or a chronically ill spouse. That is a whole different ball game. But this doesn't make the burnout we may be experiencing any less real.

I am not sure what the "magic cure" for burnout might be. But I am convinced that the problem of burnout extends beyond those who actually come down with its symptoms. It seems to me that at least part of the problem has to do with parents who *never* get involved in the first place. It's human nature, I suppose, to take for granted what you already have and are so *very used* to having. When young parents today put their children with disabilities on the school bus, it is routine and automatic for them. It probably doesn't cross their minds that without the unified push of a previous generation of parents, they wouldn't have the federal law (Public Law 94–142) that opened so many educational doors for their children. They might not give much thought to the Americans with Disabilities Act, which was passed as recently as 1990 and requires businesses and public transportation systems to ac-comodate people with disabilities. And you can almost bet that many do not realize that the public awareness of today, which translates in many ways into acceptance, is due to dedicated, focused activity by members of various disability and advocacy organizations. Organization is power, and make no mistake, our kids need that power!

And yet, there is a noticeable lack of parent involvement at all levels. Year after year, the same stalwarts—mainly parents of children who have long since graduated—end up running the fair at the school for children with special needs, or the yearly fund-raising benefit for the local ARC, because "younger parents" do not come forth to volunteer or even to join. The President of the National Association for Retarded Citizens reports that during the last decade there was a slow but steady *decline* of membership. This, of course, means less revenue and consequently, fewer programs and opportunities for adults *and* children with mental retardation. And it also means that parents who do pitch in have to spread themselves thinner and thinner, risking terminal burnout. Officials in organizations are wracking their brains trying to think of ways to bring in the "new blood" essential for any organization to survive. And they are finding it no easy task.

Sometimes I think that those of us who joined in the early struggles for research money, for better public awareness, for our kids' right to an education were lucky. We didn't have the luxury of taking things for granted because there was nothing to *take* for granted. If *we* didn't fight for our kids, who would? Well, now there is ongoing research (not enough surely), wider public awareness (still too many myths), and mandatory (if not uniformly excellent) education for children with disabilities. But what about job opportunities and community-based living options? Cute little kids grow up and become adults. What happens then? Do the parents of the cute little kids think there will automatically be job training and jobs in place when the time is right? Who's going to assure this? Public officials? Consider, then, the year the state of Maryland had a large budget surplus. Even in that year, no additional funding was earmarked for the thousands of adults with mental retardation waiting for state services, particularly for job-training programs and jobs. The money went *elsewhere*.

It seems that if something isn't of immediate concern to us, we just aren't interested. What, then, can I say to those younger parents who are so complacent about the status quo? As one who used to fidget at meetings, I would say to them that the years pass faster than you can possibly imagine and that your cute little kids will be living in an adult world a lot longer time than they spend in the world of childhood. If I scare you when I warn you that your sons or daughters may well sit home for years with nothing to do, then *good!* I hope I *do* scare you. Because that dismal prospect is a reality for many thousands of adults with mental retardation. And *now* is the time for *you* to be doing something about it.

Meanwhile, a funny thing about burnout. Just when I had started to feel I didn't want to hear one more word about Down syndrome, mental retardation, and all the rest, Ben came along and gave me a hug.

I needed that!

# The Group

. . . . . . . . . . . . . . . . . . . . .

The summer he was twenty, Ben gave a pizza/swim party at our community pool. Although a few kids were out of town, we managed to round up four of his close friends to join us on a late Friday afternoon when the pool was not very crowded.

After swimming and consuming what looked to me like a life-time supply of pizza, the group went up to the basketball court. Allen and I settled in chairs near the picnic tables to watch them.

They didn't play a genuine game, or shoot baskets in any particular order. But as we watched, we realized that in some way each of them was making sure that everybody got a fair turn to throw the ball. I can't explain how they did it; it was very smooth. Somehow they managed to make sure that no one was left out. And, as always, they cheered for each other when something good happened—in this case, someone sinking a basket, raising their arms in a sign of victory!

I took pictures—some when they were in the pool standing on their hands under water, legs sticking up at various angles. They looked pretty good, but I don't think they'll be getting any offers from synchronized swimming teams. I've got pictures from the basketball court, too—the ball flying through the air, and Laura, Mara, Paul, Craig, and Ben suspended in leaps and throws.

Looking at those pictures and remembering that day at the pool, I think about how fortunate Ben is, and the others too. True, they have mental retardation; their options are limited. But in one area, they are not limited at all. They are rich beyond the experience of many of us *in the way of friendship*. It is not just casual acquaintances they have acquired, but friends, bonded and true; in a spiritual sense, together forever.

Ben's friendships seem doubly lucky because we live in the Washington, D.C., metropolitan area. Our section of the nation is well known for its very transient population: here today, gone tomorrow. But for some reason, most of the people we know have stayed right here. What this means, of course, is that Ben and many of his friends have been together for a number of years, some since they were toddlers. They've gone through school together, socialized together, and cheered for each other at Special Olympics. They've commiserated with each other about failures, real or imagined, and congratulated each other on graduating, getting jobs, or becoming aunts and uncles. They've shared many joys, and they've shared deep grief. As a result, they *know* how to *nourish* friendship. And friendship is a primary aspect of their lives.

A few years back, this stalwart group of friends was chosen to be among the first students with mental retardation "mainstreamed" into our local public school system. There were nine in the class: one youngster with cerebral palsy, two others with some brain damage. The rest had Down syndrome. They started off together in elementary school and had a very successful couple of years. The class included Craig, Laura, Mara, Meg, Julie, and Ben. Paul, whose academic ability was quite high, had been "mainstreamed" into a different school a couple of years earlier, but he maintained close social contact. After two years in the elementary school, most of the class was transferred to an intermediate school. Mara and Julie, however, remained behind because they were almost a year younger than their classmates.

The following year, all were reunited in a junior high school. They were overjoyed to be together again and to welcome several new-comers. At this school, they were integrated with the student body for various activities. But for academics and homeroom, they had their own special ed teacher, a gifted, dedicated teacher always ready to go to bat for "her kids."

She needed to be gifted and dedicated, for she more than had her hands full! Junior high school, a world unto itself; emotions up, down, and sideways. (If I had kids in junior high again, I'd leave town!) Our kids, like their "normal" peers, were a part of this environment. Overnight, it seemed, friendships turned into something more. Several romances bloomed (in the cloakroom yet)! And despite the often touching goofiness of these adolescent yearnings, their feeling were pretty powerful as they had the added dimension of years of deep and true concern for one another.

I'm not exactly talking about sex here, although there was certainly an element of sexual awareness present. The class, in fact, had taken sex education; most of us parents had insisted that our youngsters take such a course. Our kids knew the anatomical differences between men and women, where babies came from, what families were all about. They had discussed dating and its ramifications. They pretty well understood the basics. What I am talking about, though, is *romance*, complete with hugging, hand holding, whispering, blushing, giggling, a little kissing, birthday presents, phone calls, and *caring*.

All of a sudden there were couples. Laura decided that Manoj was her "date," as she called him. Manoj was one of the new classmates, a handsome boy with Down syndrome whose parents came from India. When Laura makes up her mind, it's pretty hard to turn her down. Manoj was snapped up before he knew what hit him.

Out of the blue, Craig and Meg—who'd known each other for years—became an item. With Meg so quiet and demure, Craig took on the role of her protector.

And then there were Ben and Julie. They had met as toddlers, but had not really gotten to know each other until elementary school. There must have been something about that junior high! From the day that school began in the fall, Ben was smitten. He wrote Julie's name all over his notebook and on all his homework papers, and he stated outright that she was his "sweetheart." Every afternoon after school they'd talk on the phone. She'd call him "Baked Beans" and he'd call her "Hot Dog" and they'd laugh at their own silliness. But Julie was level-headed, too. If Ben got too silly, she'd tell him to shape up . . . and he did. Nobody's ever gotten Ben to toe the mark the way Julie could. "Do your homework, Ben!" "OK."

There was a touching innocence to this romance. Ben and Julie did not *date* in the ordinary sense. Ben, of course, did not drive, so they couldn't go off alone on a date, although the time was coming when they were perfectly capable of being dropped at a movie together. In fact, "double dates" were envisioned, possibly with Craig and Meg. But for the time being, they were content to talk on the phone, see each other at school, and socialize at parties—and there were plenty of those throughout the year.

One of the biggest and most eagerly anticipated parties was Mara's annual birthday bash. Mara's parents enjoyed entertaining the whole class, along with other parents and friends. They would have a great cookout and Mara's dad would take the kids on rides in a big wagon attached to his tractor. Then there would be a magician. The kids always loved this, especially when the magician would ask someone to come forward to be his "assistant." Once Julie was the one to be handed a "magic wand." Ben almost melted with pride.

Ben's own birthday party was another momentous event and Julie's name always headed the invitation list. On several occasions, we held the party at a combination pizza parlor and games arcade. I remember riding in the car with Julie and listening to her discuss the various games to be played there. She had a real understanding of the whole setup, and was very articulate in explaining it. Try as he might, Ben could never beat Julie at any game, and, in truth, I doubt that he wanted to.

Other kids' birthday parties often included bowling, followed by a stakeout at a pizza parlor. Here Julie was at a slight disadvantage. As are about 40 percent of children with Down syndrome, Julie was born with a heart defect, a severe one. Even after several operations . . . and facing more . . . her lips and fingertips were tinged with blue. Once in the cafeteria some students asked her if she'd been eating blueberry popsicles. They weren't being cruel; it was an honest question. They hardly believed her when she said no; her blue lips puzzled them. To Ben they were beautiful. In fact, Ben thought brown-haired, brown-eyed Julie was the prettiest girl in the whole school.

The heart condition exacted a high price. Physical exertion—especially climbing stairs—took its toll. "Wait for Julie, she's still on the stairs!" As often as not, one or more of her classmates would slow down to walk with her, and that *one* was always Ben.

The dictionary defines the word "plucky" as *marked by courage*. That was Julie. She never let her physical frailty get in the way if she could help it. At parties, lifting the bowling ball and carrying it to the throw line was a big effort, but cheered on by her peers, Julie would do it with a flair, and likely as not with a strike!

Julie did a lot of things with a flair. Academically she was at the top of the class. She read beautifully and even though Ben was handing in papers with Julie's name all over them, the teacher never confused Ben's messy scribble with Julie's neat and precise work.

One day the teacher noticed that Julie seemed crestfallen and near tears, very different from her usual demeanor. When questioned, Julie announced, "I want to be a cheerleader!"

Why not? The teacher acted immediately . . . some inquiries, some negotiations . . . becoming a co-sponsor . . . and not only Julie but others in the class became members of the Pep Squad which cheered at all the home football and basketball games. They proudly wore their blue-and-yellow tee shirts emblazoned across the front with the school logo, a wild stallion, and personalized with their names on the sleeves. And no member of that squad cheered with more school spirit than Julie and her classmates! Ben went to a few games, but his school bus schedule made it difficult to remain after school unless some complicated driving arrangements were worked out ahead of time. When he couldn't get to the games, Julie gave him a full report by phone, and this seemed to satisfy both of them.

All in all, the junior high school years were good years, and the interplay between our kids and the regular student body was pretty smooth, if not overabundant. A few of the "normal" kids even volunteered to act as tutors—a great experience for all involved.

One morning, though, something happened which had the whole school talking. Mara was returning to the classroom when someone grabbed her pocketbook, ripped the strap from her shoulder, and made off with it. Mara, who is known for her collection of pocketbooks and notebooks, did not take lightly to this theft. She hollered for the teacher, and the two of them sprinted down the hall and apprehended the thief! The purse snatcher turned out to be a student who had stolen before and even had a minor record. Mara had to talk to the police, identify the culprit, and make a formal complaint. She did it without blinking an eye, and became something of a school celebrity. "Don't

Mess with Mara!" Her classmates were extremely proud of her, and in a kind of reflected glory took on the stature of a group to be reckoned with.

After two years in the junior high, the class moved to a senior high school and into a work-study program. Everyone was excited about this step and considered it a very grown-up move. And it was. Part of the day was devoted to academics and the other part to jobs out in the community. This was real job training and it included learning to make change, use public transportation, use a public phone, cope with an emergency (what if the bus doesn't show up?)—any practical experience which could be used to enhance future job possibilities.

In the classroom there were discussions: what to do if you got on the wrong bus, what to do if someone were mean to you at work, what happened if you had to go to the bathroom, suppose a stranger started talking to you at the bus stop or tried to get you to ride in a car, etc., etc. Though Ben and his friends were no longer together all day long, they were still a cohesive group, mutually supporting each other, encouraging one another, rejoicing in each individual's success.

It was well into fall and the school year was moving at a good clip. Some of the kids were already placed in jobs, some were about to begin, others were working at jobs within the school while waiting for jobs in the community. The class would begin the day together in homeroom and then the members would bid each other goodbye and go off to their various job sites. Before dismissal in the afternoon, they'd return to school in time for some socialization, a part of the day they all looked forward to. Meeting up before the school buses departed was an important part of the routine, for often the kids took turns going home with each other. The kids always seemed to get a kick out of riding a friend's school bus, and of course the parents were grateful that this worked out so well because it saved yet another jaunt by car.

There was a settled comfort to the whole school routine, but also a sense of anticipation. Halloween was coming and everyone could hardly wait! The class buzzed with holiday preparations. What are you going to be? A witch? A monster? A candy bar? We're having a Halloween party!

One Monday morning in October, Julie did not come to school. This was not too unusual because health problems often kept her at home. And she was not alone. Some of the others also frequently missed school, struggling with bronchitis, respiratory ailments, even pneumonia. Sometime during the week, though, the teacher called—as she always did when someone was absent more than a day or two—and found out that Julie was in the hospital. At that point, the doctors thought she had a virus, probably a kind of pneumonia because there seemed to be congestion in her chest. But no one was really sure. For the present, only the family could visit.

The kids were sorry to hear this, but Julie had been in the hospital before. What bothered them the most was that they figured the virus had probably given Julie a bad stomach ache and they all fervently hoped she wouldn't have to take yucky-tasting medicine.

On Friday afternoon when they were gathered in the classroom before the school buses came, they decided to phone Julie at the hospital to tell her they were thinking of her and to get well and hurry back. The teacher called hospital information and was given a direct number to Julie's room, but the phone rang and rang and nobody answered. Disappointment was overwhelming until somebody got the idea that Julie had probably been sent home. Yes, that was it . . . and maybe she'd even be back in school next week. None too soon for Ben! On this note of hope they wished each other a good weekend and made for their buses.

Saturday the word got around. Meg's mother called toward evening. "I've got very bad news," she said. "Julie died yesterday afternoon in the hospital. It was her heart—there was nothing the doctors could do."

That gallant little heart . . . didn't make it this time . . . impossible to believe . . . her parents, how can they bear it? Ben, oh Ben, you've got to be told—no way to protect you from this . . . Julie . . . Julie. . . .

Ben was sitting on his bed listening to records. He hates to be disturbed when he's doing this; it just made it so much harder to tell him. "There's some really bad news—you're going to have to be very brave. Julie didn't make it, Ben. She died yesterday in the hospital."

"Oh no." Ben's voice was a whisper. "No—no." He bent his head slowly . . . so slowly . . . down to his chest and he stayed that way not saying another word. He accepted no comfort; he was gone, unreachable. Wanting to hold him, we left him alone.

A memorial service for Julie was held the following Tuesday. Parents, students, teachers, friends gathered to remember her. Julie's picture and a bouquet of fall flowers were on a table at the front of the church.

The service was one of simple eloquence emphasizing the joy of Julie, a celebration of her life. It was very much geared to her young friends and classmates, a remembering which they could hold to until ready to let go. The music included "Somewhere over the Rainbow," one of Julie's (and all the kids') favorite songs.

At the end of the service, people started filing out, all except the kids from Julie's class. They continued to sit, as if something were not quite finished. After a while Ben got up and walked forward to the table. He stood alone for several minutes staring at the picture of Julie, his shoulders visibly starting to sag. Pretty soon Mara quietly went up, patted him on the back, and put her arm around those sagging shoulders, and Laura followed and put her arm around his other side. Then Meg and Craig came over to give Ben a loving pat, and they all stood together as always . . . saying goodbye to Julie.

# Balance and Choices

. . . . . . . . . . . . . . . . . . . . . . . . . . . . . . . . . . . . .

One recent Saturday we drove Ben and his friends Mara and Paul out to a local dinner theater to see a revival of "Annie Get Your Gun." They were meeting fellow members of "Confidence Bound," a club for young adults with mental retardation run by the therapeutics section of our county recreation department. This program is a strong focal point in the social life of Ben and his friends, and they love it! Attending the performance and the buffet lunch preceding it (which, according to Ben, was more than worth the price of admission), is but one of many age-appropriate activities provided by "Confidence Bound." Members attend dances, visit the Smithsonian and other museums, tour the beautiful aquarium in Baltimore, go on overnights in the country, and spend weekends at Williamsburg or the beach. They do things other young adults do, but with one big difference: they do these things under supervision.

Often we drive Ben to one of these weekend functions, or to the drop-off point if the group is going on a trip. Many times we take turns with other parents getting them there or bringing them home. To tell the truth, we kind of enjoy it—even though ferrying Ben here and there is the kind of obligation most parents of grown children without disabilities can forget about. Being with Ben and his friends is often a real charge.

Right now, our transportation duties are the easy part of the balancing act we engage in as parents of an adult who has mental retardation. Most people would think of an *adult* as someone who is fully developed and mature. (A great part of the general population probably does not measure up to this standard, but that is philosophical debate for another time.) There is no way that we can honestly say that Ben is fully developed and mature. So what is he? He is certainly not a child, although he has many childlike qualities. For example, one night he asked me if I had ever heard of a bald-headed witch, and while I was thinking it over he went on to tell me that one had stopped by the house when I wasn't home and asked him for a treat, a McDonald's cheeseburger. I'm pretty sure he was putting me on—he was eighteen at the time. But I have serious doubts that this is the kind of conversation most mothers have with their adult children.

If Ben is not an adult and he is not a child, what is he? The answer has got to be that he is part of both, or both are a part of him. He is an adult, but not an adult; he is a child, but not a child. And what this means is that as his parents we are constantly trying to find the right balance—always treading that line between treating him as a dependent child and an independent adult.

We *like* having Ben at home. For the most part, he's fun to have around. I think he keeps us young! But often it's tough to keep our balance. We are of necessity involved with every aspect of his life. How, then, do we offer him the opportunity to function whenever possible as an adult rather than a perpetual child? How do we keep from intruding on the very essence of him as a person because, in all practicality, he depends on us for almost everything?

There are no easy, pat answers to these questions, no magic formula. But the one essential ingredient, it seems to me, is *flexibility*. There are times, for example, when it is *essential* to make Ben do something he does not want to do, and times when it might be better to let something go. You have to play it by ear.

"Normal" teenagers and young adults can make choices about their own lives. We may not always agree with those choices and we may even have some input concerning them. But for the most part, normal young people can choose where they want to work: McDonald's, a car wash, Pop's Pizza, a movie theater, a dress shop. They can set their own social life, and expand it greatly by getting a driver's license. They can choose whether or not to go to college, when to leave home, when and whom to marry, and whom to vote for.

Ben will make few such choices. He has a job he likes very much, but *he* didn't choose it. *We* found it for him, filled out all the applications, got him the necessary ID, took him for the required medical exam. We did the choosing.

Ben will not get a driver's license, likely will not marry, and will not vote. There is no way Ben could ever legally drive a car, and if you saw the way he drives the bumper cars at the beach boardwalk you would consider this very good news. There is no realistic way he could consider marriage. Voting is yet another matter, and here again *we* made a choice, admittedly with a touch of sorrow. Like other adults with mental retardation, Ben has the legal right to vote. But he would have absolutely no idea whom to vote for: issues and candidates would be completely over his head. Allen and I believe that someone who goes into a voting booth should know what he or she is doing and understand what the process is truly about. We also know that an unscrupulous person could easily take advantage of Ben in urging him to vote one way or another. We thought long and hard before we made the choice *not* to register him.

Even "Confidence Bound," which means so much to Ben and which he has certainly chosen to join, would not be possible for him if we did not go along with his choice and obtain the membership application, fill it out, send in the membership fee, and provide the transportation.

Because Ben's choices *are* limited, we do try to find ways for him to make as many for himself as possible. His passion for shoes is legendary, for example. He loves high tops and sports shoes of all kinds and we allow him to get a new pair almost every month and choose whatever style he wants. He's making good money, which we have to manage (Ben's math ability is at a very simple level), but it is *his* money after all. He's not going to spend it on cigarettes, beer, or cars, so why shouldn't he buy something he really enjoys? At the same time, he's not much interested in dress shoes. We insisted, however, that he buy at least one pair of those too, and after much grumbling he picked out something suitable. He hardly ever wears them, of course, but he does own them.

Ben also selects a lot of his own clothes. Our daughter Ann, the one who inspired the slogan, "Born to Shop," is great about taking Ben on shopping sprees. With her guidance, he picks out clothes *he* likes.

We are deeply grateful for her willingness to do this because shopping is not on our list of favorite things to do. *We* were *not* born to shop.

Ann is also the one who introduced Ben to "hair styling." We used to take Ben to the local barber shop, but a couple of years ago Ann took him to one of the fancier salons to be "styled." Ben was duly impressed and especially liked having a pretty woman working on his hair and fussing over him. Now he won't consider going anywhere else, and that's fine with us.

We also allow Ben to spend his off hours pretty much as he likes, which is listening to records in his room or watching TV down in the rec. room. If we go someplace, even a fun place which you'd think he'd like, he rarely wants to go with us. We'd have to drag him, so why force him? Surely he can make the choice to stay home if he wants to unless there is some absolutely essential reason that he go. We know that he sometimes misses out on things by staying home, but we think it's more important that he have the opportunity to choose. We've been letting him make this choice since he was about fourteen, and so far no harm has come of it.

To further complicate the balancing act, parents must not only encourage good choices, but also discourage bad ones. In other words, we are required to discipline someone who is of a chronological age to be disciplining himself. How do we do this? We cannot discipline him in the same way we would discipline a little kid; he's *not* a little kid. What's more, every situation is different; the outcome often unpredictable.

Sometimes Ben can be so rigid and stubborn! We usually try to avoid confrontation because that always makes a situation worse. Ben does not know how to handle confrontation; it makes him belligerent. But if given time, he usually comes around. When he has done something wrong, he invariably will apologize on his own. If possible, we try to let this maturity of his rise to the surface and help him to cope—sometimes a lot easier said than done. Here is how a typical duel between the adult and child sides of Ben evolves:

Almost as sure as the sun rising each day, every afternoon at five our phone rings. It is Ben's good buddy, Craig. He and Ben always have the same conversation, which makes no real sense to anybody but themselves. Ben returns Craig's call at five thirty—not five twenty-nine, not five thirty-one. *Five thirty!* Now, goofy as these phone conversations may be, they do allow Ben to have some control over his social life. He also talks on the phone with other friends, but not at any set time. Unless it interferes with others using the phone, there is no reason Ben can't call his friends if he wants to.

But suppose someone *else* is using the phone? What happens if Ben and Craig find a glitch in their routine?

One afternoon I happened to be on the phone with my daughter-in-law at *five thirty* when Ben wanted to make his call. He threw a fit, actually picked up the receiver of the phone extension in his room, and started yelling. I immediately cut my call short and stormed into Ben's room, intending to disconnect his phone and forbid any calls to and from Craig for the rest of the week. I had fire in my eyes, and for a minute, so did Ben. But Ben is no dummy. He saw that I was very upset with him, that I meant business and his transgression was not something to be taken lightly. This was Big Trouble! I saw the expression on his face change from stubborn, childish anger to keen awareness and he raised his hands in supplication. "I'm sorry, I'm sorry!" Lucky for him my mechanical abilities are zilch and I didn't know how to disconnect the phone. This was fortunate, for about half an hour later Ben came to me and apologized again. He then asked if he could please call his sister-in-law and apologize to her, which he did. "I'm sorry I was rude; I'm really sorry."

The next day, Ben mentioned the incident and said again how sorry he was. He promised not to act like that any more. Should I have gone full steam ahead with the punishment? Strict disciplinarians might not agree with me, but I don't think I should have. I think I handled it the right way, being flexible enough to let Ben's maturity take over. I'm *glad* I didn't disconnect his phone, or rip it out of the wall as I was sorely tempted to do. And I didn't banish Craig's phone calls either!

But another time, another situation? That will be a whole new ball game, and one in which we *might* have to step in, however reluctantly, and allow Ben *no* leeway. Do we or don't we? Should we or shouldn't we?

Allen and I are the parents of four. Three of our children grew up. One did not, exactly. He is a beloved son, and more than anything we want to do right by him. Often when we are dropping Ben off or picking him up at his various functions, we stop to chat with other parents. Over the years many of us have shared a lot of comings and goings. And we've shared more than that. All of us are striving for balance. We live with children who are not children, adults who are not adults. Choices. . . . What's right? What's wrong? What's neither?

We were not trained to walk the balance beam with skill and grace. We can only do our best and hope that it is enough.

# Average

. . . . . . . . . . . . . . . . .

An article I read in a Sunday supplement has really set my teeth on edge. It was written by a mother verging on desperation in trying to find the "right kind" of private preschool for her three-year-old son.

Apparently the competition for admission among brightly normal preschoolers is putting their poor parents into a pressure-cooker situation. According to this mother, one school required—among other things—a "self portrait" from her child. Can you blame the woman for having the vapors when the poor little tyke's best efforts produced something resembling strands of tangled, colored spaghetti?

In addition to asking for the applicant's strengths, the applicant's weaknesses (be reminded these applicants are between 2 and 5 years old), recommendations from family friends, parents' philosophy of education, etc., many schools set up a "test" with an educational consultant. The test lasts about an hour and parents are not allowed to be present. Not only that, this parent who paid the eighty-dollar test fee was not told the test results. She found out something else, though. A prestigious school in New York State came to the conclusion that the tests were putting undue pressure on children who were barely past babyhood and the tests were inaccurate in predicting potential. Get this: the school reported that children who showed great promise at age three became, in its parlance, "disappointingly average" at age five.

Disappointingly Average!

These "finest schools" and frantic parents are having to deal with kids who are *average*. The kid may not wave bye-bye until he's a year instead of ten months old, might not walk at nine months as the neighbor's prodigy did, might not talk "early," or be toilet trained before three. And the poor child may not learn to read until the *end* of first grade rather than at the beginning or even before. The list of things the average child will do at less than accelerated speed is endless. Now, it is very natural for parents to be proud of their children, to extol their virtues whenever they get the chance. I'm not faulting anyone for that—goodness knows I'm guilty too, and, in fact, when it comes to our baby grandson, I have great difficulty keeping my mouth and my photo album shut.

What I find so disturbing—infuriating really—is what the concept of average has come to mean in certain circles. Average has become a dirty word, an undesirable quality, an anathema to be avoided at all costs. No better example of this attitude exists than in those schools described by this mother seeking placement for her three-year-old, and, I fear, in the mother herself. It is very obvious that the kid who won't be Phi Beta Kappa in kindergarten is counted out. Average is simply not good enough; the child who is only average is less worthy of being accepted into a prestigious school, *preschool* at that, and if the child is less worthy, what does that say about the *parents?* The time of year when private preschools send out their admissions decisions is absolute torture time. Anxious parents must wait to find out if their three-year-olds have made the grade, and thus, if *they too* have made the grade.

Where does this leave those of us who most certainly do *not* have this problem of average to worry about in our children with mental retardation? One thing for sure, it leaves us free (or should) of a dreadful kind of myopia. If you have a minute, look up the word *myopia* in a dictionary. The definition which I find meaningful is *a lack of foresight or discernment; a narrow view of something.* Those who suffer from this kind of myopia are simply unable to see just how extraordinary "good old average" can be.

Through the years I have observed that most of us who have a child with Down syndrome also have "normal" children. This gives us a unique opportunity to daily witness the state of being average. It also gives us—or should—a certain equanimity when our normal kids don't win the most beautiful baby contest or show early promise of being a ballerina, a high-school football star, or a Rhodes scholar. We don't hit the roof when they bring home report cards bearing C's instead of A's and B's. It's not that we don't want them to have special talents, make top grades, or be highly successful. Rather, it's that we understand the *value* of average. If Ben had ever brought home a genuine C in arithmetic, or anything else, we would have been overwhelmed, literally jumping with joy all over the house.

This brings to mind that old saying about not really understanding someone until you've walked a mile in that person's shoes. It may be that it is just not possible for those hung up on the "anathema of average" to understand how many of us are able to accept average with aplomb—well, almost.

Here I should note that although most of us can readily appreciate average in our "normal" kids, some parents cannot do the same for their kid with Down syndrome. On the one hand, they find it easy to disparage those who seemingly worship the elitism of the upper percentile. On the other, they cannot accept that their child be any less than a super-achieving kid with Down syndrome. They spend every waking hour trying in every way they know to milk that last ounce of potential out of their child. It's one thing to put great effort into enhancing opportunities for your child. It's another to become obsessive about it and think of little else. Sometimes it seems that while it is OK to be average/normal, to many parents it is not OK to be average/retarded. . . . there's a double standard.

I guess what it boils down to is this: each of us wants the best for our children, all of our children—super, average, not-so-average. We who have kids with Downs know what it is to leave no stone unturned in our efforts to enhance opportunities for them. We can't in fairness look askance at other parents who do the same for their own.

But I have to be honest. Fair or not, those who label a child "disappointingly average" *still* set my teeth on edge.

# Every Parent's Nightmare

. . . . . . . . . . . . . . . . . . . . . . . . . . . . . . . . . . . . . . . . . . . . . . . . . . . .

This is not an easy subject to write about, and I've spent a lot of time trying to find the best way to approach it. I've decided to just come right out with it. We have reason to believe that Ben was sexually molested while at work. It happened a couple of years before graduation when he was still participating in the school work-study program.

Here's the worst part: we did not find out about the incident until *one year later*, and then only by a fluke.

Today, after the fact, I believe our antennae would pick up the signals; Ben's actions would certainly alert us. Back then, however, we just didn't get it; we didn't know a thing until it was too late.

In retrospect, perhaps we should have known something was going on. And, believe me, we have anguished over it. Were we stupid or what? I still don't know, and that's the main reason for sharing our experience. If even one parent is forewarned and can prevent something similar from happening to another child, the discomfiture of writing about Ben's experience is worth it.

One Monday morning, Ben didn't get up for school. He stayed in bed moaning and groaning and complaining of a terrible stomach ache. I checked him out, and although he looked OK and had no fever I took him at his word. This is a kid who loved school, got himself up every morning, fixed his own breakfast, and walked down to the corner to catch the school bus. His routine was as reliable as the rising and setting of the sun. He *never* wanted to miss school.

As the day progressed, he seemed better, even got dressed and sat on his bed playing records. He also ate lunch and dinner. It was just a bug, I thought.

But the next morning, Ben was moaning and groaning again and wouldn't get out of bed. I let him stay home—one more day, I decided—and by afternoon he seemed fine.

Wednesday morning it was the same scenario, so off to the doctor we went. She examined Ben and concluded he was generally healthy, but that his stomach was very tense, almost spastic. She prescribed some medicine to relax his stomach and said he could go back to school in a day or two.

I let him stay home the rest of the week. By the end of the weekend, he seemed perfectly fine, but on Monday morning he refused to get out of bed. "Ben, the medicine has helped you," I said. "You've got to go back to school."

"I won't—I won't go back!"

What was I supposed to do now? I couldn't force him out of bed and drag him to the corner to catch the school bus. I was really upset. Something was very wrong and it was definitely more than a stomach ache.

Later in the day I called Ben's teacher to tell her what was going on. She racked her brains trying to think of anything that might have happened at school to upset him so. Nothing came to mind, but she said she'd talk to the other students and see what she could find out.

That night, feeling pretty desperate, I went in and sat next to Ben on his bed. "How are you feeling?"

"OK."

"All your friends miss you very much. Would you like to go back to school tomorrow?"

"No!"

"Ben, is something bothering you, something you haven't told us about?"

It was almost as if a shadow passed across his face and he looked at me, and looked away. Then, in a very low voice, "Timothy hit me."

"Hit you? He hit you?"

"Timothy hit me in the stomach and he called me bad names." His face was troubled; surely he was not making this up. But what he was telling me didn't exactly make sense—or did it?

Timothy was not another student, someone who might possibly have picked on Ben at school. He was a member of the maintenance crew at the shopping center where Ben worked every morning as part of his work-study program. This particular job site was highly valued because the management of the shopping center had been very cooperative and permitted several students to work there at various hours during the week. Not all area businesses are so enlightened. In addition, the kids had less than a five-minute walk from school to get there.

Up until this minute, we had thought Ben was very happy on the job. He had mentioned Timothy once or twice, but with no particular emphasis. On the contrary, he had talked about his boss, Brett, with enthusiasm and admiration. Much to Ben's pleasure, Brett had even given him a Christmas present. The only thing I knew about Timothy was that when Brett wasn't there Timothy was the *one* in *charge*, whatever that meant.

I called the teacher to report what Ben had told me. She immediately got in touch with the job coordinator—the person responsible for finding the students jobs in the community—and the two of them went to talk with Timothy and Brett. Timothy denied Ben's allegations, said Ben was a nice kid and he wouldn't want to hurt him. Brett backed him up; he had never seen any signs of trouble, not with Ben nor anyone else.

Ben stuck to his story. And he adamantly refused to return to school. But obviously, the problem was not school: it was the job. More precisely, it was *Timothy*—whether for real or imagined reasons.

To say that we were truly confused and did not know *what* to think is an understatement. Was Ben telling the truth? Ben is not one to lie, but he does have a lively imagination. Was Timothy telling the truth? Was it some kind of giant misunderstanding that would never be resolved?

At length we reached a compromise. Ben's work hours were changed so that he would not have to be on the job when Timothy was there. Apparently Timothy only worked part time, so this was easy to arrange. Their paths would never have to cross again.

In looking back, it seems kind of odd that Timothy didn't question this arrangement, since in a way it was an affront to his innocence.

We'd been told he was low on the socio-economic ladder. Maybe he didn't want to rock the boat and risk losing a job he needed.

At any rate, it was essential that Ben get back to school. We presented the plan to him. "You won't ever have to see Timothy again."

"For sure?"

"For sure!"

"OK!"

He returned to school and the job the next day and was immediately caught up in his comfortable routine. He never mentioned Timothy's name again and there was no sign that he was disturbed in any way. To all appearances he was the same old Ben.

Almost a year passed. Ben no longer worked at the shopping center. He was now in the "Big Time," the Bethesda Naval Hospital, the prestige job site where all the kids longed to be assigned. Here he worked in the kitchen, sorting silverware, loading and unloading the huge dishwashers, stacking trays, and doing whatever else he was asked. He loved his job and was very proud that he had learned to take public transportation to get there.

One day Laura entered the classroom with a startling announcement. "A man touched me on the shoulder when I was on the bus!" What this might—or might not—mean was anybody's guess. But it did create the opportunity for a class discussion.

The teacher, assistant teacher, and all the kids gathered in a circle. Laura explained how she was returning from her job to school, on the public bus, not the school bus, when a man had touched her. Whether this was accidental or intentional was unclear, but the incident opened up a dialogue on "good touching," "bad touching," private parts, etc. It was then that Ben dropped his bomb! He stood up and said, "Timothy made me pull my pants down and he touched me." The teachers just about fell to the floor. They were totally stunned. They weren't the only ones.

After the discussion ended, the teacher called me to relay what Ben had said. I could hardly believe what she told me. Neither could Allen when he came home from work.

Parents' fears for their children are universal, of course. Whether or not those children are small or grown up, normal or disabled, we still have fears for them, particularly when it comes to sexual exploitation. When our children have mental retardation, our fears are often compounded because our kids are so trusting, so terribly vulnerable. We can tell our kids, any of our kids, about "sex," and schools can do the same, but we cannot with surety protect our children from every situation that may arise. Apparently, such an unforeseen situation had caught up with Ben. And remember, the person Ben had accused was not the *lurking stranger* offering candy or other goodies, but someone he knew, someone who was an authority figure to him . . . someone he had trusted.

Is it any wonder our first reaction was shock and confusion? We really did not know what to do, what first step to take. One thing we did know was to avoid putting any kind of pressure on Ben. Secure in the company of his friends, Ben had felt free to let go of a bad secret after hearing Laura relate a similar experience. At least that's how it appeared to us. We did not press him, but we gently asked him about what he had told the kids at school. He repeated his story to us and then he didn't want to talk about it anymore.

We set up a conference at school. The two teachers, the job coordinator, the head of the jobs program, the superintendent of special education, and a school psychologist were there along with Allen and me and our daughter Ann, who insisted on coming. Ben was not present. All of us felt the meeting would upset him greatly and his presence would possibly inhibit a frank discussion.

Here is what we found out at the conference. Everyone was sympathetic to Ben and concerned about any possible emotional damage to him. BUT: at the time of the alleged offense, Ben was eighteen, barely, but eighteen nevertheless, and therefore not a minor. Did this mean he was a consenting adult? I guess so. And how many times had it happened? Once? More than once? Ben himself couldn't seem to say. In addition, the alleged offense—offenses?—had taken place a year before, and no accusations had been made until now. Ben seemed to be fine, and no other kids on the job site had complained of similar incidents. Moreover, when it got down to the nitty gritty, it would be Ben's word against Timothy's. If it went to court, would a mentally retarded person's testimony carry the same weight as a non-retarded person's? *Above all*, would we really want to put Ben through the trauma of a trial and everything *that* entailed?

Timothy, of course, was denying that anything had happened. The teacher and job coordinator had gone again to the shopping center to see him in the presence of Brett. The two said Ben had made the story up; Brett backed Timothy to the hilt. Weeks later we found out that Brett and Timothy were in-laws, but at the time of the conference we did not know this. And I'm not sure it would have made any difference if we had.

What Allen and I had to decide was whether or not to pursue legal action. Uppermost in our thoughts was WHAT IS BEST FOR BEN? Do we let it go and try to forget about it or do we press charges knowing full well they probably won't stick? This was one of the most traumatic dilemmas we had ever faced in raising Ben.

I wish I could tell you that we solved it satisfactorily and with peace of mind. We didn't. About the only thing I *know* we did right was to insist that parents of kids then working at that job site be told what had happened—what possibly had happened—to Ben. A couple of parents allowed their kids to remain there; others had their youngsters transferred to other jobs. Other than that, we have always been left with a vague feeling that we didn't do something quite right, that we goofed up in some way. Maybe we let the school system off too easy. I think school officials were afraid we were going to sue, but that was the last thing on our minds. If that guy had really molested Ben, we wanted to *get him*; simple as that.

In the end, we really did nothing. We did not go to court, we did not even go over to the job site and confront Timothy, which had been our first impulse. In fact, Ann and Claire, gentle, tender-hearted girls, were ready to go find Timothy and "punch out his lights!" So was Douglas. It was not easy to talk them out of this, but we pointed out that if we went to court, pummeling Timothy could only hurt Ben's case. I couldn't blame them, though. I had the same urge. I was physically ill for days after hearing about Ben's experience and I have no idea what I would have done if I'd been face to face with this man.

The bottom line is that we will never know for sure whether Ben was molested. We believe that he was. Whatever happened, it apparently left no permanent scars. Although Ben is reserved with strangers (nothing new about that), he's good at making and keeping friends. He's always had great rapport with teachers, counselors, bosses, and co-workers. He's never been withdrawn or depressed, nor shown any signs whatsoever that something deep down is disturbing him.

We consider ourselves lucky.

If given the chance would we handle things in a different way? . . . Probably.

To begin with, I hope I would recognize that when someone as routine-oriented as Ben suddenly breaks that routine, *something is wrong!* I hope I would take nothing for granted, not even a stomach ache. I hope that if given that second chance I could help Ben sooner. Hindsight, of course, makes us wise.

Secondly, I wish we *had* pursued legal action, at least to the point of consulting a lawyer. It's not that we doubted then—nor even doubt now—what school officials told us about our chances of winning the case. But I just wish we had talked to a lawyer.

Lastly, distasteful and sickening as the thought is, Allen and I should probably have confronted Timothy. Not with Ben—he would never have gone—but just the two of us. At the time, we were advised to let the school authorities act as go-betweens, and we agreed. Truthfully, after my initial reaction of wanting to do Timothy bodily harm, I really could not bear the thought of seeing this man in the flesh. Allen felt the same way. What were we afraid of? That we would see in his eyes that Ben's accusations were true?

I hope with all my heart they weren't, but. . . .

*Graduation is certainly a time of mixed emotions. Nostalgia, pride, and concern for the future are all part of that very special milestone in the lives of our children. No parents are more attuned to these feelings than those of us who have children with disabilities. This essay was written on the eve of Ben's graduation from Walter Johnson High School, Bethesda, Maryland, held at the John F. Kennedy Center for the Performing Arts, June 1988.*

# A Joyous, Painful Graduation

The voice on the phone asking to speak to my son sounded efficient, yet friendly. Call it a mother's instinct if you will, but I *knew* he was a recruiter for the armed forces.

No surprise because Ben's name is on the list—make that *lists*. As a graduating senior, for months he's been hearing from the Army, Navy, Air Force, and Marines. It happened that Ben—or Bennett, as the voice referred to him (no doubt from a list)—was not home, and when I told him this he wanted to know when Bennett would be back.

I asked him outright if he were a recruiter and he said, yes, he was a recruiting sergeant for the Army.

Moment of truth. Even after all these years it is not easy to inform a stranger that my son is mentally retarded. But it seemed only fair to let the fellow know he was wasting his time trying to recruit Ben. "Sergeant, there's something you should understand. My son, Ben, has Down syndrome; he is mentally retarded."

A slight pause. "I'm sorry to hear that, Ma'am," he said, and it was obvious from his tone that he didn't believe me; another over-protective mother trying to keep her baby boy from the clutches of Uncle Sam.

Ah, Sergeant, if you only knew. All those brochures touting "The opportunities in today's armed forces are better than ever!" ... But not for the likes of Ben.

Graduation. Another young adult about to go out into the big world . . . or is he? After the "Pomp and Circumstance," the parties, the gifts, the signing of the yearbook, what then? Come September when his fellow graduates go off to college or enter the work force or follow the sergeant's call to arms, where will our graduate be?

The bitter-sweet nostalgia of graduation time brings tears to many eyes. My eyes will have tears, too, when I see Ben march to pick up his special education diploma, but my tears will not be flowing from the well of nostalgia. It's more likely they'll be tears of fright and apprehension, of being downright scared at what might happen to this decent, sweet, capable young man when the school bus doesn't stop at our corner any more.

Perhaps it's those brochures that have skewed my view of this particular graduation. The Army letter, for example, tells Ben: "You can choose from hundreds of occupations and get skill training for a lifetime . . . and starting pay of $573.60 a month before deductions. . . ." The Marines promise him "skills that can help you to get a job . . . or move ahead in the job you have." The Air Force wants to help him grow "through experience and education" and is willing to pay 75 percent of tuition for off-duty civilian courses.

Last summer I drove Ben to the post office where he was required to register for Selective Service. The postmaster was friendly and kind and there was compassion on his face as the two of us watched Ben avow his name and sign the necessary form in what we knew was a futile action.

The irony of Ben's being the recipient of all the brochures is that the job training they stress is *exactly* what he needs. He'll never design a computer program, learn accounting, or fly a jet aircraft. But there are jobs he could do—and do *well*—if he had basic, solid, intensive training.

Ben already has proven he can function in the working world. Part of his school curriculum has included working at various jobs in the community. He has been a member of a cleaning crew in a shopping center, folded towels and linens in a motel laundry, been a busboy in a cafeteria, even worked as a kitchen helper at the Bethesda Naval Hospital.

In all of these positions he received some minimal on-the-job training. But like most retarded persons who have a real job potential, Ben needs thorough grounding in what it means to develop initiative, motivation, productivity—vital attitudes and skills employers prize in any worker.

Most so-called normal people pick this up on the job, as do some retarded persons. Ben has partially done so and has performed passing well in his various jobs. The consensus, however, is that Ben needs a no-nonsense, intensive work-training program for about six months to make him truly ready for competitive employment.

Ben is not alone. Others graduating with him have the same need, and graduates going back five, six years and more, still are waiting to hear they've been accepted into a work-training program, waiting and losing what skills they possessed at graduation time.

It's great to see pictures of the Special Olympics, to read about the family that adopts a dozen retarded children, to watch a movie about the cute retarded kid who melts everybody's heart. The fact is that at local, state, and national levels there isn't enough money to provide work-training programs for many young—and not so young—retarded adults who *need* and *want* to work.

Society seems willing enough to help foot tuition for youngsters going off into the armed forces or to college. But if parents cannot afford to pay for job training, their retarded children are often on waiting lists for months, years, and in some cases, forever.

Parents, then, are forced into a kind of terrible game trying to outwit one another in proving the desperation of their situation. Those parents who succeed might get funding and their child will get job training.

We'll celebrate Ben's graduation from Walter Johnson High School June 5. With other parents we're planning to hire a limousine to have our special graduates arrive in style for dinner at a fancy restaurant. And there'll be a party, family and close friends, music, dancing, gifts, and somewhere along the way there'll be pizza—to Ben how can there be a celebration without pizza?—and we'll have photographs, hugs, and congratulations. It will be a glorious day, a day to remember, always.

Ben recently heard from the Army again. They sent him a poster, a huge one to put on his wall. It's a copy of that famous poster from World War I; a stern, compelling Uncle Sam points his finger at the viewer.

I WANT YOU. I almost wish.

# Smart/Dumb

. . . . . . . . . . . . . . . . . . . . . . .

If someone were to ask you what most often surprises you about your son or daughter, what would you say? If Allen and I were asked that question, we would say it's that Ben can be so sharp and so dumb in almost the same breath. Sorry if the word *dumb* offends, but I'm stating it as we see it. Thinking about this rather fascinating personality trait of Ben's sent me back to the dictionary to look up the word *dichotomy*. Dichotomy is defined as: "a division or the process of dividing into two mutually exclusive or contradictory groups." Don't you think this definition is applicable to our kids? There are many times when Ben and his friends have proven themselves to be clever and resourceful, sharp as tacks, as the saying goes. By any standards they would be members of "the smart group." But then, in almost the same breath, it seems, they can be so dense, naive, and obtuse that—and it pains me to say it—they would be consigned to "the dumb group." And we never know from one minute to the next which group will lay claim.

One afternoon after work Ben was in his room playing a Beatles album and when it was finished he came to me and announced, "The Beatles lived in the twentieth century."

"That's right, Ben," I said, "they sure did."

"But some people lived before The Beatles and that was the twentieth century and some are living now and some will live later and that's still the twentieth century. We are in the twentieth century!"

"Yes, Ben, that's very true. I think what you're talking about is the passage of time."

He looked at me and nodded his head. "Yes, that's it!" And back he went to his stereo.

Wow! Is this kid a profound thinker or what?! I felt so happy, almost overwhelmed in fact. Somewhere deep inside, Ben was really able to put it together.

A few days later Ben's friend Paul was at our house to spend the day. The boys had come in from shooting baskets when the phone rang.

It was Laura wanting Ben to go to the movies. When she learned Paul was visiting us, she invited him to go along too. The guys thought this was a fine idea!

Laura and her mother would come pick them up and they would go to one of those multi-complex theaters so the kids could attend one movie while Laura's mother attended another. Then they would all go for pizza. I had Ben and Paul check their wallets to make sure they had plenty of money to pay for their tickets and their share of the pizza, soft drinks, and snacks.

When Laura and her mother showed up, Ben and Paul piled into the car and went off happily waving goodbye.

Several hours later they were back grumbling with indignation about something and commiserating with each other.

"What's wrong?" I asked. "Didn't you like the movie?"

"It was great!"

"Then what's wrong? Did you have trouble buying your tickets?"

"No, Laura bought our tickets."

"What do you mean Laura bought your tickets? Do you mean *she* paid for them or did you give her the money to buy them?"

"*She* bought them with her own money. She *wanted* to. . . . BUT SHE WOULDN'T SHARE THE POPCORN!"

"Who bought the popcorn?"

"Laura bought the popcorn, THE GIANT SIZE, but she wouldn't share it!"

Because this is starting to sound like an old Abbott and Costello routine, let me sum up what apparently transpired at the movie theater. Laura bought all the tickets with her own money because she wanted to "treat the boys." (Her mother later confirmed this.) Laura bought the popcorn at the theater and later everybody chipped in for pizza, and Ben paid the tip. But the only thing these two incipient gigolos could think about was that Laura had refused to share the popcorn. The fact that she had paid for their tickets didn't phase them; in fact, it didn't register with them at all. The popcorn, or lack thereof, was all they could think about.

"Hey you guys," I asked, "didn't you have your wallets with you and didn't you have money in those wallets?"

"Yes," they answered with no inkling of what I was getting at.

"Well, you both had money, so why didn't you go to the refreshment stand and *buy your own popcorn?*"

Surely there was no more illumination on the day Edison "invented" electricity than in the light bulbs which simultaneously went on above their heads. They looked at me in astonishment and admiration.

"What a great idea!" Ben said.

"Next time we'll do that!" Paul said.

"Give me strength," I said.

This is one of the tough realities that we face as parents of a son or daughter with mental retardation. We see such potential in our kids, but it so often ends up skewed somehow. We may well have learned to expect the unexpected but all the same it can still cause us anguish. In a real sense we too are dichotomous. Even as we anguish, we can see the funny side. Do we laugh or do we cry? Often we do both—and, like our kids, almost at the same time.

Nobody is surprised when little children pull some funny and seemingly paradoxical stunts, exhibiting a complete and often disarming naivety in some actions even as they are precocious in others. We all have tales to tell about something "so adorable," "so funny," "so remarkable," that any one of our children—or grandchildren—has done. Grandson Tyler, a plucky little fellow, is terrified of the laundry chute in our house. (Odd how he suggested that new Baby Sister might like being dropped down it.) And when Ben was seven, he developed a positively ingenious plan to hide the fact that he'd somehow lost his brand-new glasses. Rather than admit to losing them, he kept telling us various places he'd "left" them. What a merry chase he sent us on, laughing all the while! At his behest we looked in the washing machine, the dishwasher, the garbage disposal (*that* was a good one), and all the trash cans—to no avail. Eventually I found the glasses on his closet floor, and much to Ben's disappointment, the "fun" was over.

When Ben was a child we sort of assumed that he would someday outgrow this curious dichotomy. I do not mean we thought he would outgrow having mental retardation. But we figured that with maturity the "smart/dumb" behavior would diminish, that he would be less naive, less divided, less prone to do something *really dumb*. His "smarts" would win out, at least most of the time.

Well, we now know it doesn't necessarily work that way. Ben's personality is a fusion of the two, and we have observed that this holds true for all his friends who have Down syndrome. In fact, the older they get, the more noticeable it is. I don't believe they are doing anything more outlandish than they have done previously. It's that they are no longer children, chronologically, and any aberrations in their behavior therefore seem magnified.

And still we often find ourselves taken unaware, even though we have been conditioned to expect the unexpected. I am not sure why Allen and I continue to be so astonished by what Ben and his friends do or say, but we are. Wonder and puzzlement play a large part in our lives.

Why did Laura generously insist on buying movie tickets for Ben and Paul and then refuse to share popcorn with them? What was going on in her head that prompted her to do this? (I wonder, by the way, what the other movie patrons did while the great, whispering popcorn argument took place?)

And what of Ben and Paul? Many times these two have walked to the nearby shopping center to buy themselves sodas and snacks, and every day at work Ben buys soft drinks from the vending machine. When Laura refused to share the popcorn, why didn't they *even think* to go buy their own?

Or how is it that while on the job Ben saw a customer drop her wallet and showed the good common sense to follow her to her car and politely return it (and receive a commendation from management for doing so)? Yet, a few hours later when his favorite TV station was knocked off the air by a power failure, he ranted and raved like a two-year-old demanding it go back on the air *right now*, and no amount of explaining would pacify him?

I would expect that most of us have wondered at one time or another about this character trait in people with Down syndrome. Sometimes it seems as if they are saying yes/no at the same time. I don't remember coming across a definitive, satisfying explanation for this in any of the books and articles I've read. If there is one, I'd like to know what it is, just to satisfy my curiosity. But I'm under no illusions. At this point I don't think an explanation would make any difference in our lives.

In addition to all the bewildering frustration we have experienced through the years, we have had the chance to observe the most admirable qualities in Ben and his friends, qualities to make the hearts of parents swell with pride and gratitude. We see in these young people honor, sensitivity, compassion, empathy, and a finely tuned sense of justice.

Even as we have learned to expect the unexpected we have also learned to expect the best.

# The Job!

. . . . . . . . . . . . . . . . .

Until recently, I can't say that I was ever emotionally touched while pushing a grocery cart, unless you count the time I dropped a can of cat food on my big toe. That does bring a quiver to the lips. A grocery store is, after all, a utilitarian environment. You just don't think of it as a place where lives can be affected or changed forever. In fact, you probably don't think of it much at all—unless, that is, there is a teenager or young adult with mental retardation in your family. Then you start viewing grocery stores, fast-food restaurants, shopping malls, and any number of business places with a very personal interest. Could my kid handle a job here? Would they even give him a chance?

In theory, of course, we knew all along that Ben would one day graduate from school and be faced with finding a real job. Part of Ben's special education curriculum *was* job training in the community. He worked at various places: a laundry, the kitchen of the Bethesda Naval Hospital, a cafeteria, a shopping mall. He learned to use public transportation, and he liked all of his jobs. He got along well with bosses and co-workers. Everything was fine . . . as long as he was in the public school system.

Once graduated, though, people like Ben lose options that parents of "normal" kids can take for granted: college, jobs, job training, military service. Instead, people like Ben have their names put on waiting lists, lists that often have years of backlog for even minimal job training or workshop programs. In federal and state government, funding for adults with mental retardation is not a priority. This is a sad and ever-present fact of life.

Some local communities do offer hope. In our area, for example, the local ARC works with county government and private industry on the job front, looking for employers willing to place or train people with disabilities. At the state level, however, I had encountered disaster. The year before Ben graduated, I had filled out detailed application forms requesting possible state funding for job training. After months of waiting to hear from the state office about Ben's status, I learned that the forms had been lost.

I filled them out a second time and mailed them off. Again they were lost. Outraged phone calls got me a third set but with no guarantee they'd ever be processed. Incompetence and inefficiency were the rule, not the exception, in this particular state office. Other parents I talked with had suffered the same experience—just what we needed when we were facing crisis milestones in the lives of our children.

I suppose my initial brush with this particular state agency should have prepared me for their bungling of Ben's applications. Shortly before graduation, Ben was evaluated to determine what kind of job placement would be best for him, a moot determination considering there was no money to place him anywhere. The consensus reached at the evaluation was that Ben was "too high functioning" to be in sheltered employment and would definitely benefit from job training— too bad about the money or lack thereof. What did this mean for Ben? Nothing, as far as we could figure. (Although I'm convinced that declaring Ben "too smart" was a ploy to save money in some way.) By the time his name surfaced at the top of the waiting list, it would be geriatric aid he'd need.

Eventually, we gave up any idea that the state of Maryland would ever help Ben with job training or opportunity. In a way it was a relief. No point in wasting energy on fruitless pursuits.

We concentrated on finding out all we could about job programs in our county. There were a few possibilities, some of them promising, but not for Ben as it turned out, or—perhaps more accurately—not for his parents.

During this time when we were desperately afraid that Ben might end up spending months or years sitting at home, we made a *vital* discovery. It's not just *the kid* who is involved with the job. The whole family has to live with the *hours*, the *location*, the *transportation*, etc. We hadn't really thought about this before. When Ben was in school, he went off on a school bus and he came home. We took it so for granted.

Ben wasn't the only one graduating.

In digging around, we got the feeling that some directors of job programs concentrated so much on the individual actually enrolled in a particular program that the needs of a family as a whole were not realistically considered. For example, one program required that the participants take public transportation to and from the training site. No exceptions. They were not to be driven there. I agree with this requirement in principle. But we lived three bus rides and probably two hours away—that's *each way*.

If you think about it, how many teenagers or young adults take three buses to get to work, especially at night? When their son or daughter is late, parents may chew their fingernails and glance at the clock a lot, but just the same, the kid's driving the family car, or more than likely, a car of his or her own.

Still, my attitude was not much appreciated. Worse, it eliminated an option for Ben.

In a way, though, our experience with the job training program opened up another option, for Allen and I had learned something very basic. Unless parents want to settle for a job that's less than ideal, they may have to find the job *themselves*. And because we weren't willing to settle for just any job, we decided to find Ben a job that would be best for him and best for us in *our own particular circumstances*.

We set up some basic goals. First and foremost, we would try if at all possible to find Ben a job in our *own* community. If he had to take a bus to get there that was OK, but it would have to be *one* bus and a ride of no longer than forty-five minutes.

Like many parents we know, we decided that only as a last resort would we consider seeking a job at a fast-food restaurant. We had a few mixed feelings about this decision because food service offers a prime employment opportunity for people with mental retardation. But Ben, who is already a bit "portly," loves to eat and being around all those hamburgers and french fries would be a temptation he could *never* resist! Then, too, there was the matter of schedules. A couple of Ben's acquaintances worked for fast-food chains. They had no say about the hours they were to work and often were scheduled from late afternoon until ten at night, or later. One youngster had to give up Special Olympics practice as a result. We weren't willing for Ben to do this—he needs that exercise!

We also scratched convenience stores from our list of job possibilities. It seemed to us that unsavory characters were always hanging around these stores. And, unfortunately, such stores are often targets for robbery. If Ben were to witness a hold-up, he wouldn't be quiet about it, that's for sure! Indignant and making no bones about it, he would unwittingly put himself in grave danger. No way would we risk it. Perhaps we were being overly cautious about this, but our gut feeling told us we were not.

Another consideration for us in the great job search was Allen's impending retirement. After years of arduous commute on the infamous Washington Beltway he was not anxious to take on complicated driving duty, and he was planning to begin lots of projects at home. Both of us were more than willing to accommodate our schedules to any possible job Ben might get—but within reason. We were not going to build our entire lives around "The Job."

Having set up these sort-of ground rules, we started looking. At first the search didn't have that much urgency. True, every time I went anywhere, I evaluated it as a possible job site for Ben. But at this point, I was not ready to actually go up to someone and ask about a job. Partly I hadn't gotten up my courage, and partly we wanted to enjoy summer vacation.

But then came September, and for the first time in almost twenty years Ben was not climbing aboard a school bus. It didn't seem to bother him at all, but for me it was a tremendous shock! The change put everything into focus as nothing had before. Either Ben was going to sit home on perpetual vacation or we were going to have to do something *now!*

I soon found out that despite a lot of positive publicity about hiring the handicapped, there is no plethora of jobs. There are many more people with handicaps—especially with mental retardation—who want and need to work than there are jobs available for them. And you had better believe that many people in positions of authority are still reluctant to hire someone with mental retardation, no matter how great the publicity.

You can usually tell right off if a potential employer will *never* be receptive. Phone calls aren't returned, or if they are, the person is evasive—he claims "We're not hiring now" or passes the buck to someone who's never there. If you get this kind of response, I believe you should save your energies and look elsewhere.

Other possible employers give mixed signals, maybe not even knowing they are doing so. A nursing home I called, for example, at first gave me real encouragement about Ben working in the kitchen as a *volunteer*, no pay involved. In fact, because Ben was eligible for a job coach, they'd actually be getting two workers for free!

In the spring before Ben's graduation, I had by chance made contact with the Foundation for Exceptional Children in Reston, Virginia. Under the auspices of the Foundation, a group called *Team Work* was training retired volunteers to act as job coaches for would-be workers who had mental disabilities. If Ben needed a job coach, thanks to *Team Work* one would be available for him. (A job coach is someone who goes on the job with the handicapped employee to help in any way possible, acting as a liaison between the employee and job supervisor if necessary. Sometimes job coaches are needed indefinitely, and sometimes for only short periods.) The Director of Volunteers at the nursing home seemed receptive to the idea of trying out Ben and a job coach. We talked several times and she said she would like to meet Ben after she discussed him with the owner of the nursing home. We were going to set up an interview, but when I called to do so, I got a song and dance about the kitchen workers not having time to teach Ben. When I reminded her that Ben had worked in several kitchens and had done just fine and that the job coach would be there, she said she'd call me back, but she never did.

This experience was very disheartening. What chance did Ben have if they wouldn't even meet him? The reality of Ben's retardation hit home harder than it had in years. Ben was no longer a cute little kid. He was a young adult who spent his days playing records and watching TV.

Obviously, we needed to regroup. I prepared a resumé for Ben, listing every job he had held through his high school program, every activity he had participated in, and interests such as music and sports. I wrote it in terms that presented him as someone involved with life, not as someone sitting home like a lump doing nothing. Resumé in hand, I then investigated a preschool, another nursing home, even a horse stable, and more I can't recall—but without success.

One day I noticed that our local hardware store had a "Help Wanted" sign on the door. I knew it was a long shot, but I went in and asked. They were looking for someone good with figures who could run a register—not someone like Ben—but at least they were forthright about it.

I checked out the movie theater at a nearby shopping mall, one of those multiple theater complexes. The young man I talked with was reasonably receptive. He asked me if I thought Ben could take tickets and direct patrons to the movie of their choice. I was sure he could, although it did cross my mind that if a movie Ben particularly wanted to see were playing, he'd direct everyone into that one. (I kept this to myself, of course.) We also discussed the possibility of Ben doing maintenance: sweeping, picking up trash, mopping up spills. The conversation ended on a high note, for me anyway. The fellow told me he'd talk to his boss, the theater manager, and I should call back the following week.

In the meantime, I had a hunch and called the offices of Giant Food, Inc., a large supermarket chain in the Washington, D.C., area. I asked what the policy was on hiring someone who has mental retardation, and was told it was up to the manager of each store. In retrospect, I've concluded that this sums up our kids' chances of success on the job: Up to the Manager!

It happens that we shop at Giant, and have for years. The following Friday evening while we were doing our weekly shopping, I gathered my courage and knocked on the office door. I told the kindly looking woman who opened it that I wanted to speak to the manager. She informed me that *she* was the manager. I was so nervous that I just blurted out, "I need a job!"

At the time, I was wearing my Daffy Duck sweatshirt and my red sneakers splotched with paint, so when I explained it was not for me but for my son with Down syndrome, I think she was relieved.

Those of us who have children with mental retardation can be the best advocates in the world. That isn't enough, though, unless people in the community will meet us halfway—no, more than halfway—to give our kids opportunities. I had found such a person. She listened with patience to my frantic pitch. When I was through and expecting to hear that they'd like to help but didn't think it would work out, she told me she'd give Ben a chance and handed me an application. It took every bit of restraint I could muster not to jump up and down in my funny red sneakers.

She went on to explain that she and her staff would do all they could to help Ben and to teach him on the job, but two things would be necessary for Ben's success. One, we would need a job coach. Two, Ben would have to have the right attitude. His cooperation and willingness to take orders and work with others would determine his job future. If it worked out, he would be paid better than minimum wage and he'd be required to join the United Food and Commercial Workers Union.

The *Team Work* Program Administrator, Tillie Walden, arranged for a job coach, who met with Ben and got to know him before the job started. It took almost a month to complete the paperwork, fill out the application (too complicated for Ben, so we were allowed to do it for him), get a T.B. test, and obtain a copy of his birth certificate. A little friendly advice here: Ben needed I.D. similar to a driver's license. When our other kids had gone for licenses, a copy of their birth certificates had sufficed. But now we needed one embossed with the official state seal, or in this case, a seal from the District of Columbia, where Ben was born. This meant a trip to the office of vital statistics or a six-week wait. Allen went to the office in person and got it the very same day.

The long-accepted pronged T.B. test wouldn't do, either; it had to be a drawn blood test. We found this out *after* we'd had the pronged test done. Poor Ben, back again. In fact, we hustled like crazy to expedite every requirement. I felt almost driven, so afraid that there'd be a hitch or that somebody in the company would decide against hiring Ben after all. I couldn't forget the nursing home fiasco.

Ben started working part time at Giant in October, four months after high school graduation. The job coach, a gentle, patient, retired psychologist named Harvey Taschman, helped Ben for two weeks. By then it was apparent that Ben didn't really need a job coach anymore. Store manager Barbara Dougherty and Mr. Taschman both felt that Ben could take directions perfectly well from store personnel. (I'm happy to report here that the Dole Foundation for Employment of People with Disabilities, established by Senator Robert Dole in 1984, has since awarded the Foundation for Exceptional Children a grant to continue its *Team Work* program.)

Ben's official job title is Courtesy Clerk, not exactly what we call him at home. His primary duties are loading groceries into customers' cars and keeping shopping carts in order. On Mondays, he does inside work ripping covers off unsold magazines. (He excels at this, but we haven't figured out if this is good or bad.)

Would you believe that this store is only about five minutes by car from our house? We settled quickly into a flexible routine. Allen or I drive Ben to work so he is always on time. If it rains or snows, one of us picks him up. He can also take a bus if he wants to. But he loves to walk home and will soon be walking *to* work as well. In fact, he walks on a bike path through the woods. This route allows Ben to indulge in a favorite quirk. He is crazy for sticks, twigs, and branches, so when he comes through the woods, he brings part of the woods home with him. That's why the front of our house looks as if a woodcutter lives here, why it's decorated with a sort of Hansel and Gretel motif. Allen periodically gathers up a load of kindling and returns all he can carry to the woods, but Ben just brings home a new supply. We try to consider it a form of exercise for both of them.

Shortly after Ben started working, I had a revelation of sorts. I had assumed that once he got a job I could relax about it. Instead I became obsessed with trying to find out how he was doing. I didn't dare rock the boat by being obtrusive and asking outright. So I took to spying on him from various locations in the shopping center: from behind cars in the parking lot, leaning against a support pillar near the store entrance (hoping I looked casual), positioned between the trees bordering the complex. Allen warned me that I might be taken for a robber casing the joint or an industrial spy from another grocery chain. He also expressed the opinion that the dark glasses and Orioles baseball cap I wore pulled down over my ears were not all that great a disguise (although he did concede that I bore a vague resemblance to a short Gomer Pyle). One day a policeman approached me as I leaned against the pillar. *This is it* I thought, but he passed on by and went into the Chinese carryout. And as often as not, Ben spotted me and made it clear that he didn't like my being there at all. But I *had* to know.

I did observe that at first Ben was very slow, picking up one bag at a time to put into a car. (I wanted so much to run over and help him.) But I also noticed that most people were very patient with him. This was a good sign. It also touched me to see Ben wave goodbye to every customer, even when no one waved back. One thing surely stood him in good stead. We belong to the swimming pool which borders on the far side of the shopping center. Many of the pool members shop at Giant, so a lot of customers know Ben by sight if not by name. And some of these people went to the manager and told her how pleased they were to see Ben working there.

Eventually I gave up spying and Ben speeded up considerably at his job. He works independently now at the loading zone and he's been given other duties as well—for example, loading up the candy and drink machines, dream duty for sure. His fellow workers are very fond of him and have taken him to Baltimore to see the Orioles play. In July 1989, Ben was named Staffer of the Month at his store. What impressed him most about this was that he and the honored staffers from other stores were treated to a great breakfast!

This job is probably one of the best things that's ever happened to Ben. Every night he gets his clothes ready so he can put them on first thing in the morning. He watches the time and knows when to leave and always remembers to bring his time card. He is not able to figure out his finances in any detail, but is proud that he himself is now earning the money to buy his shoes, clothes, albums, and wrestling magazines.

He *likes* the responsibility of the job and feels a duty to be there, no matter what the weather. In the almost three years he has been at Giant, he has rarely missed a day of work, except to go on vacation.

But it goes beyond just him. Allen and I have also benefitted. It is an enormous satisfaction to us to see Ben succeed. Now we know that he is able to hold a job and that he is capable of being at least semi-independent. His earnings are nothing to be sneezed at either. The cost of his various activities—camp tuition, for example—no longer comes out of *our* budget. Best of all though, we have found Ben to be his most mature self when he is on the job.

Others, too, are touched and hopefully influenced. Ben is recognizably retarded, no doubt about it. And there he is every day functioning responsibly in a very busy, *visible* community setting. What better statement that hiring the handicapped works?

A door was opened for Ben. When a door is opened for one, it can be opened for others. Who knows what prospective employer shopping at Giant might be given food for thought—no pun intended—simply by seeing Ben on the job?

The other morning I dropped Ben at the store, parked the car, and went in to do some light shopping. As I was rounding an aisle with my cart, I chanced to see Ben greet the assistant store manager, his immediate supervisor, with a big grin and a wave that were promptly reciprocated. Ben looked so happy, so self-assured and mature. There was an aura about him, a sense of belonging. He didn't stop, but moved on to his duty post without spotting me.

I stayed where I was for a minute, pretending to look at the pickles and olives. It's better not to push a grocery cart when your eyes are full of tears.

# Unbidden Shadows

. . . . . . . . . . . . . . . . . . . . . . . . . . . . . . . . . . . . . .

One thing about having a child born with Down syndrome or any other handicapping condition is that you never look at a pregnant woman in quite the same way again. In the back of your mind there is always the question—I wonder if the baby might be. . . ? We can look at a stranger and hope things will be OK for her and then go on about our business without much further thought.

But what if the pregnant woman is someone we know, someone we love? A sister? A daughter-in-law? Our own daughter?

Families that do not include a child with a handicap may consider the possibility that something could go wrong, and then dismiss it as too negative, too remote to dwell upon. But the knowledge that something really *can* go wrong looms frighteningly large once it has happened.

I cannot speak for someone else. I do know that Allen and I would be very apprehensive if we were young parents again and were expecting a baby after having had Ben. And I know, too, that we would avail ourselves of any and all tests that would tell us if it were going to happen again.

Does this raise a question that none of us even want to admit asking? No matter how deeply buried or unacknowledged our feelings, do we resent our child with disabilities because the very fact of his or her birth has made any subsequent pregnancy a scary proposition? Even though chances are slim that it would happen again, there will always be a certain uneasiness. Pregnancy is now overshadowed by a dilemma. Do you have the test and possibly be faced with a terrible choice? Do you forego the test and sweat it out?

No matter what you do, part of the charm, wonder, enjoyment of pregnancy is lost forever. Our rational minds tell us that if something goes wrong it's nobody's fault, but does that make it any easier to deal with? All those long years ago when Allen and I were raising our young family, the idea that someday we might become grandparents and have new concerns seemed so far away. Although sometimes I tried to imagine what it might be like, the realities of today usually cut such imaginings short. After all, becoming grandparents only happened to "old" people. (Boy, have we changed our point of view on that one!) And certainly, in those far years ahead, how we would feel about the impending birth of a grandchild had nothing to do with Ben. We were too busy worrying about today, and in truth, scared of tomorrow, at least where Ben was concerned. How would he turn out and what would happen to him? Those were the questions we were asking then.

It is pretty overwhelming to realize how fast the years have flown. It is even more overwhelming to know that in a couple of months Allen and I will become grandparents for the second time. Our daughter Claire, the one we thought destined to become the world's oldest practicing cheerleader, is expecting again. We are delighted; can hardly wait, in fact. We have so much fun with grandson, Tyler, and now we get to double the fun! It's the excitement akin to anticipating a wonderful new gift. But as with Claire's first pregnancy, there's this nagging little worry in the back of our minds which keeps the joy Allen and I feel slightly out of focus.

No matter how many times we remind ourselves that we already have a perfectly beautiful, button-bright grandson and will probably have another grandchild just as bright and beautiful, we are not at ease, and won't be until we know everything is OK. Claire chose not to have the pre-natal testing the doctor suggested because she has a sibling with Down syndrome. To be candid, I wish she had done it. I would have. But I did not urge her to have the test or even express my opinion on the matter, except to tell her that it was up to her. This was not easy, I confess. (I certainly have no hesitation informing people that such tests exist—and have done so.) But having pre-natal testing is such an intimate, personal decision for a married couple to reflect on—and so are any options that may follow. It is certainly not up to Allen and me to tell Claire and Gregg what to do. And it is most definitely not up to the government to tell them what to do either!

At the time the doctor suggested that Claire undergo chorionic villus sampling, done much earlier than amniocentesis, Claire said to me, "I love Ben; I can't even imagine what our lives would have been without him. If it happens to us I think Gregg and I could handle it."

I was very touched by her words and proud of her, but in my heart I am a realist. Being raised as the brother or sister of someone who has a handicap, particularly a mental handicap, imparts uncommon insights, true. Nevertheless, *it is not the same as being a parent with all the responsibilities of parenthood.* I hope they could handle it. I also hope with all my being that they will never have to.

Our older son, Douglas, was married recently. And in time, our daughter Ann may well marry. (A mother can hope!) Each time a grandchild is on the way, the wonder, the looking forward, the just-can't-wait excitement will be tempered with apprehension and the knowledge that things *can* go wrong. We've noticed, though, that friends who've become grandparents and don't have a child with handicaps in their family don't seem bothered by such thoughts. I suppose their equanimity is related to that attitude that it only happens to somebody else, never us.

But it *did* happen to us and it changed forever the way we look at things. A baby is born with Down syndrome and from then on every pregnancy in the family reflects that baby's birth in heart and mind. Feelings which touch each generation are evoked: fear, sorrow, joy, relief, anger, exaltation, dread.

Is it going to happen again?

I don't think we can definitely resolve these feelings. Possibly the best we can do is just accept the fact that they exist. In no way do they detract from the love we have for Ben. They are simply part of the package of having a child with Down syndrome.

We look at the pregnant stranger and wish her well. We look at our daughter and can only hope that soon we will see her holding a normal, healthy baby. Only then will those old, haunting feelings subside, at least for a while.

# A Touch of Reality

· · · · · · · · · · · · · · · · · · · · · · · · · · · · · · · · · · · · · · · · ·

The other week I heard some bad news. It was Ben who told me, his eyes sad and worried. "Vickie Victory has been poisoned!" I drew a total blank and stared at him, uncomprehending. I wasn't even sure I'd heard him right. Was someone he works with gravely ill? Those troubled eyes looked to me for some kind of response and I struggled to think of something to say to him. He gave up on me and repeated, "Vickie Victory has been poisoned." Then he added, "The Woman in Black did it!"

It came clear in an instant, and I had to turn away. I could not look at that anguished face and laugh, so I bit my knuckles, took a deep breath, and turned back to him. "Gee, I'm really sorry to hear about it, Ben. I hope she'll be all right."

"Yeah," sighed Ben, "but it's very serious," and he left the room.

Now, lest you think I am callous and lacking in sympathy for the unfortunate Vickie Victory, let me explain. Both Vickie and the Woman in Black are female wrestlers, part of those great Show Biz extravaganzas on TV. Ben is but one of many caught up in the hyped and scripted showdowns between the good guys and the bad, the heroines and villainesses. There are literally thousands and thousands of TV wrestling fans as enthusiastic as can be, knowing all the while that these are staged morality plays.

To Ben they are not staged at all. You will never make him believe that all the posturing and boasting and sneaky slams are acting (actually, very cleverly choreographed). To Ben this is *real*. He believes it as a small child believes that Santa Claus visits every house in the world on the same night.

Is it any wonder that parents of kids with mental retardation are split right down the middle? The humor of various situations, a certain skewed way of looking at things, is so downright funny you would have to be a rock not to laugh, but oh the problems your endearing innocent can bring!

Many people still equate mental retardation with unmitigated stupidity and the antiquated term *moron*, and single out those who have it as the butt of dreadful jokes. Parents of children with Down syndrome know that this image—one to make us grit our teeth—is far from the truth. Our kids may not excel in academics, but stupid they are not! In many areas they are perceptive, knowledgeable, clever—sometimes *too* clever. Yet, there is no denying they must face life with a large disability, disparity, gap—call it what you will.

What is the single most limiting factor in Ben's having Down syndrome? If someone were to ask me that question, I would answer that it's not that his math ability is zilch (he *can* work a calculator), that his reading is at the third-grade level, that his version of history is oddly garbled (you should hear him explain the demise of Thomas Jefferson), that physics and engineering and computer science, etc., etc., will be forever beyond him.

The most limiting factor in Ben's life is his lack of sound judgement. And it is this curious lack which makes him so vulnerable and, therefore, disabled. Through the years some of his judgement calls have been and continue to be memorable—his insistence on wearing eight pairs of sweatsocks at one time; his habit of tying his shoelaces so tight that by day's end his feet are almost purple; his passion for collecting sticks, branches, and tree limbs which he keeps piled near our front door; his multiple and oh-so-silly phone calls to and from his friend Craig, and Ben's inability to end the conversations even when they clearly bore him.

These actions of his often add to the funny part of our family tapestry, but not always. Sometimes they just leave us sort of bewildered. Take the morning Ben forgot his uniform cap when he went to work. His Dad, who'd driven him, told Ben to go in and punch his time card and he'd be back with the cap. When he returned, there stood Ben waiting in the same spot. Ben had not entered the store because *you do not punch your time card and report for duty if you are not wearing your hat!* That goes against the routine. It did not occur to him that his presence on the job with or without his hat was what was important here. In many ways Ben is so sharp that this behavior threw us a curve. Is this what having mental retardation truly means?

Not too long after the hat incident, I had a phone call from a friend who has a fifteen-year-old son with Down syndrome. Her call almost jolted me out of my socks, and yet I was so grateful that she'd made it. (What would we do without other parents?) It seems that an acquaintance called and told her of seeing a young man with Down syndrome working at a supermarket. His job was loading groceries into customers' cars. She observed that during the lull between cars he was talking to himself. From the location described, I knew right off it was Ben. Not only was he talking to himself, he was saying, "Damn it! Damn it!" (Oh, why does he have to have such clear speech?)

But wait, it gets worse! As the woman was about to go into the store, she noticed Ben look sort of stricken, grab himself, and wet his pants. I'm not sure what the shopper did, but I went into absolute panic on hearing this bit of news.

Did she report Ben? Did anyone else observe him? What would happen if they found out at the store? Should we go to the store and talk with someone? Should we keep quiet and hope no one else knew about it? Was Ben going to get fired?

My friend had called on a Friday. Allen and I spent the whole weekend trying to decide what to do. (Ben does not work on weekends.) The job has been so great for Ben and he loves it. The thought of his losing it had me in tears.

As we considered various options, we gradually realized what Ben had been up to. His active imagination had been at it again. He had taken his passion for wrestling to work with him and was pretending to be different wrestlers—his heroes from TV. "Pow!" "Take that, Pal!" "You're gonna get it now—Doomsday!" All this in front of the grocery store. Although what Ben was doing was clear to us, to strangers his behavior could well seem bizarre, even frightening.

The reason he wet himself wasn't hard to figure out either, an almost damned if you do and damned if you don't situation. A courtesy clerk, someone who loads groceries into customers' cars, is not to leave his duty post unless it is covered by another employee. Ben understands this, maybe too well. It is obvious he was caught in a terrible dilemma exacerbated by the soft drinks he buys when on his break. Because he's not always good at anticipating, that lack of judgement again, he doesn't think to use the bathroom while on his breaks, especially when the drink-vending machine is uppermost on his mind.

What to do? Is there a solution? No doubt, but we're not sure yet what it will be. And there's another consideration that will have to be handled with great finesse. Sometimes it seems as if Ben's feet are set in concrete, the famed stubbornness of the Down syndrome personality. Our older daughter, who has great rapport with Ben, has pointed out something we hadn't thought too much about. Because she and Ben are of the same generation, she probably understands him a lot better than we do, and her insights about him make a lot of sense. Ann believes that Ben doesn't act the way he does just to be stubborn per se and not because he has Down syndrome. She says he simply wants to make his own decisions and to be independent, just as other young adults do. He may not know how to go about it in the same way, but it doesn't make his longing for it any less valid.

So now we've got our work cut out for us. If we are at all confrontational in telling him that he must stop acting out his wrestling fantasies, and that he *must remember* to go to the bathroom, he will probably resist us, at first anyway. This is nail-biting, hair-pulling frustration, for we know he understands the difference between appropriate and inappropriate behavior, but again it's lack of judgment getting in the way. The worst thing we can do is to yell at him, or lecture him that if he doesn't shape up he may lose his job.

No, there's got to be another way to go with this. To paraphrase what Jack Benny used to say—we're thinking, we're thinking.

Meanwhile, I get so tired of walking on egg shells and sometimes so angry inside—not at Ben, but at the circumstances, and that means the attitudes of others that must be dealt with. I know I'm not the only parent of a son or daughter with mental retardation who's fed up with bending over backwards to preserve someone's sensibilities or to woo someone's approval of his or her child.

Why do we keep doing it?

There is so much concern these days about mainstreaming, community living, "normalizing," and indeed, most of us are involved in trying to achieve these very goals. But somewhere along the way is it possible we've slipped up? Are we so intent upon making society accept our kids in all the normal settings that we've forgotten something very basic? Although Ben has many normal attributes, he is *not* normal. Ben has mental retardation and no matter how much we may wish otherwise, this is a fact of life.

Do not misunderstand. I am not making a pitch here for inappropriate behavior, but maybe I'm sticking up for something akin to *affirmative action*. Parents should not have to panic if their kids goof up. But we do. For my part I know it has to do with the thousands of adults with mental retardation whose names are on waiting lists for jobs and job training. The idea of Ben's losing his job and spending his days waiting and waiting for something meaningful to do scares the hell out of me!

I do not know why that customer called my friend to tell her about the boy with Down syndrome whose behavior was less—a lot less— than exemplary. (Admittedly, this is not a sight anyone expects or hopes to see when embarking on the weekly grocery shopping!) Perhaps it was a genuine concern so my friend could be forewarned about her son's potential behavior. I like to think that this was the case, but I'm dubious. I'm not even sure why.

For a year now Ben has had great success at his job ninety percent of the time. Most people have been wonderful, accepting, and even joyous to see Ben working there. Some have taken the time to go to the manager and express congratulations that Ben was hired. Still, we are on the defensive and I hate it. I hate thinking someone will see him at work and be turned off, so turned off they might report him.

I can understand that it doesn't exactly make for a happy shopper to see the courtesy clerk talking to himself and wetting his pants smack dab in front of the supermarket. But after all these years, I understand too that inappropriate behavior is often part of the reality of mental retardation. The shopper faced it as a single incident (we hope!). We face it as a life-long challenge, and right now part of that challenge is to buy enough time for us to work with Ben to eliminate his faulty behavior. If only a complaint isn't made against him.

Ben will shape up. He generally comes through if given the time and lots of patient understanding. We're counting on it, and we're still thinking.

Oh yes, some good news. Remember Vickie Victory? Ben reports that she has fully recovered and that she flipped out the lights of the Woman in Black!

# "Charles"

. . . . . . . . . . . . . . . . .

Sometimes I think that Ben is less than a drop of DNA away from being a genius. I am not saying this just because Ben is my son and I am proud of him. I'm saying it because it seems a logical conclusion when viewed from a historical perspective. Think about it. Throughout history, geniuses have been noted for their eccentricities and idiosyncracies. Consider, for example, the poetess Emily Dickinson, who secluded herself in her father's house and for almost thirty years never left it. Or Mozart—a divinity in the world of music—whose money habits and antics in the presence of his royal patrons were nothing short of bizarre. And what of Thomas Edison, Alexander the Great, Leonardo da Vinci? (Did you know that Leonardo was not only ambidextrous but also wrote his notes backward with his left hand and then read them in a mirror?)

It wouldn't take much effort for any of us to come up with a list of geniuses whose behavior would certainly be considered as strikingly out of the ordinary. Now, whether or not these "quirks" manifested themselves before or after the genius was recognized as such, I don't know. I haven't really delved into the fine points of this and I'm not sure it matters. All I know is that if *unusual* behavior is one of the hallmarks of being a genius, then I am not wrong in believing that Ben is right on the edge.

Although Ben is no stranger to unusual behavior, it was not until the summer he was twenty-three that I glimpsed his true genius. It was three weeks or so before swimming season ended for the year, and Ben and I were up at our community pool. I was floating around in the deep end wishing summer would last forever when I noticed Ben climb up the ladder and stand at the edge of the pool. I saw him sort of arch his back and thrust out his belly, looking down at it with obvious admiration. Then he patted it lovingly and I thought I saw him talking to someone, or something. I had never seen him do anything like this before and I didn't really know what was going on. I let myself sink to the bottom of the pool, hoping no one else had noticed his decidedly weird, but oh so funny actions. When I came up for air, Ben was headed for the basketball court which is part of our pool complex. I stayed in the pool until it was time to go home, and, to tell the truth, forgot about the incident—but not for long.

The following weekend, Ben and Ann took the subway downtown to spend the afternoon and have lunch at the Smithsonian Museum of Natural History, a place Ben dearly loves. They were gone for hours. When they finally arrived home, they were both worn out but said they'd had a great time. Ben was impressed with the dinosaur exhibit, which Ann had particularly wanted him to see, but as always his main thrill was viewing exotic masks from Africa and South America. And of course, lunch!

After Ben reported the day's events and went upstairs, Ann said to me, "Something really strange happened." I wasn't sure I wanted to know, but I told her to go ahead and lay it on me.

"Well," Ann said, "after lunch Ben stood back from the table and pulled up his shirt and talked to his belly."

Just what every mother longs to hear. "And what did he say?"

Ann looked at me kind of funny. "Are you all right?"

"I'm fine. What did he say?"

"He patted his belly and then he said, 'Charles.'"

"'Charles'?"

"Yes, he called his belly 'Charles' and he sounded exactly like a persnickety English butler when he said it."

"Are you telling me he has a belly named 'Charles'?"

"That's what I'm telling you, Mom."

"And he talks to it?"

"He certainly was talking to 'Charles' in the cafeteria because I asked him point blank what he was doing and ordered him to pull his shirt down at once, and he told me he was talking to 'Charles.'"

It seems that those who went to the museum that day got more of an exhibition than they might have hoped for!

I can't help but wonder what Dear Abby or Ann Landers would advise in this situation. As experienced as they are, I'm not sure that even *they* would come up with any answers.

I think I've figured out the reasoning behind "Charles," but what to do about it (him) is something else. Like many people with Down syndrome, Ben is too heavy—at least we think he is. He is five feet and one inch tall with broad shoulders and muscled arms, a naturally husky fellow, and he has great legs (like his father and brother!). Ben might well have been a six footer and played football on the high school team if things had been different. But thoughts like these are little help in this situation. I'm much more concerned with the excess weight in that belly of his which he is so adamantly attached to, no pun intended. Ben knows we want him to lose weight, but he won't even consider such heresy. My guess is that he has invested "Charles" with a personality in order to protect "him." I doubt that Ben *truly* believes "Charles" is real, but if the creation of "Charles" doesn't show genius, I'd like to know what does! How many people do you know who could come up with such a unique plan?

And it seems that thus far we are not equipped to deal with someone who is functioning at genius level, at least in this one area. We offer no solutions. If you are contending with a similar problem, we cannot help you. Alas, we cannot even help ourselves.

As of this writing, Ben continues to nourish "Charles" and encourage his growth and expansion while we do everything we can think of to diminish "Charles" and cause him to disappear altogether.

So far, Ben and "Charles" are winning hands down.

# The Spectrum

...........................

When Ben was about fifteen, our family doctor suggested a physical examination and evaluation to check for problems that can sometimes arise in adolescents with Down syndrome. She recommended that we take Ben to the Down Syndrome Clinic at the University of Maryland School of Medicine in Baltimore. Because Ben's friend, Mara Paulson, was referred to the clinic at the same time, her mother, Rae, and I drove them there together.

The clinic was not crowded that day. When we arrived, there was one family with a baby not yet a year old. The baby, a boy, was cute and lively, and the young parents were full of hope for the future. They played with the baby and proudly listed his accomplishments. They seemed eager to talk with Rae and me and asked us a lot of questions about Ben and Mara. Rae and I were happy to oblige, and when a nurse came to get them we were all so busy talking we didn't even notice her.

No sooner had they gone off with the nurse when another couple came into the waiting area. They too were accompanied by a boy with Down syndrome, but not a baby. This boy appeared to be about the same age as Ben and Mara, maybe a year or two younger. It was hard to tell. The youngster walked very slowly and didn't seem aware of his surroundings at all. The parents led him very carefully to a chair and helped him sit down before they themselves sat down next to him.

At first the parents didn't say anything, but I noticed that they were both intently watching Ben and Mara, who were having a lively conversation about all the toys and books piled on the floor in the middle of the room. Coming to the clinic was nothing to be sorry about for these two kids. In addition to getting a day off from school, Rae and I had promised them lunch at Baltimore's wonderful Inner Harbor if we got out of the clinic in time. They were in high spirits and the toys and books were an added bonus, even though they eventually decided these particular toys were for "little kids."

As the parents continued to rivet their attention on Ben and Mara, Rae and I looked at each other with silent understanding. We both wanted to say something to them, but what? It was obvious they were intrigued with our kids. I knew instinctively, and so did Rae, that it was the alertness, the liveliness, the verbal give-and-take between Ben and Mara that had so caught their attention.

Finally I asked the most mundane question I could think of. "Where are you from?"

It turned out they were from a small town in Pennsylvania and they had come to the clinic, as we had, to have their son examined and evaluated. Once the ice was broken, they opened up to Rae and me. Their son was sixteen; he went to a school for the mentally retarded not too far from where they lived. He did not speak, did no academics, and had trouble walking. Within the last year he had been toilet trained. The parents did not belong to a parent group and knew of none in their area. They had also never seen any other kids with Down syndrome, except those who went to their son's school and were apparently on the same developmental level as he was.

When they asked where Ben and Mara went to school, Rae and I were almost reluctant to admit that our kids had for years been in regular schools, albeit within their own special-ed classes. And we did not tell them that Ben and Mara could read and write, although I'm sure they realized it from observing them.

All the while these two parents were watching our kids and talking with us, their own son sat, not moving, not saying a word, still showing no interest in his surroundings. A sorrowful knot formed in my stomach, and I knew Rae was feeling exactly the same. Our eyes met. What could we say to them? What could we do? And each of us was thinking—Boy, are we lucky!

Then it was time for Ben and Mara to go to their respective appointments. Shortly thereafter a nurse came for the boy, who walked slowly away supported on both sides by his parents.

That visit to the clinic which is imprinted so vividly in my memory raises a question. How do parents who have such high hopes for their kids—kids who are achieving many milestones—deal with parents whose kids are lower functioning and achieving very little?

What Rae Paulson and I felt that day was not new to us. Through our parent group, we had spent time with kids with Down syndrome, babies and older, who were not keeping pace with other kids with Down syndrome. We had seen the faces of parents who were braving it out, knowing that their children were not only children with Down syndrome but were lower functioning than most other children with Down syndrome. And our understanding went deeper than that. As parents of kids with Down syndrome who function in the "average" range, Rae and I had more than once seen our kids suffer in comparison to what I call the "Super Down Syndrome Kid."

Who is the Super Down Syndrome Kid? He is this era's answer to the barely-functioning Mongoloid—a wunderkind who can do everything almost on a par with "normal" kids. Although the two are poles apart, they share one unfortunate similarity, I believe. They are both unrealistic stereotypes. Where *are* all the Super Down Syndrome Kids, anyway? I think of all the youngsters with Down syndrome I have known—and there have been many—and I can recall no one who has achieved "super status." I am talking about someone who can participate *totally* in a regular school curriculum (even tempt fellow classmates to copy from his or her homework assignment), someone who attends college doing *bona fide* college-level work (not special courses), someone who has developed the skills necessary to make it in an office job as more than a gopher—who is able to do intricate filing, sorting, typing—someone who could be a truck driver, a store manager, a full-fledged TV or movie star. I don't personally know a single individual who has approached such achievements.

I don't see this as negativism. I see it as reality. Think about it. In the spectrum of abilities, where do most people with Down syndrome seem to fit? Consider those you know, children and adults. Wouldn't you agree that most are somewhere in the middle or perhaps *slightly* toward the high side of the spectrum? They all have their own strengths and weaknesses, as does everyone. Some are sharp in one way, not so sharp in another, but generally most people with Down syndrome are *average* Down syndrome people. This certainly means they function very well, are capable in many areas, and lead happy and productive lives. But they are *not* super achievers, and no matter how much effort we put forth on their behalf, they never will be. The majority of us are not going to end up with a "Corky" of TV fame. The majority of us will end up as parents of a son or daughter who is in or near the middle of the spectrum. And that's OK—better than OK, in fact!

Now, what about the *lower* end of the spectrum? What about those who not only have no hope of being a Super Down Syndrome Kid, but won't even be an average kid with Down syndrome, no matter what parents do? More to the point, what about those parents? Where do they turn when they need someone to talk to? Do they turn to parents of the Super Kids? Do they turn to parents of the average kids? Do they perhaps just turn away?

I think we have a dilemma here. Of necessity, we must set our sights high. One thing for sure, if we don't, nobody else will. Society as a whole isn't going to gratuitously give our kids a leg up, especially in hard economic times. We *have to* paint a positive picture. The great reality is that most people with Down syndrome do very well when given opportunity. We know that; our job is to make sure that others know it too. In order to gain that opportunity, we *need* the "good press." We *need* to publicize success—the mainstreaming stories, the jobs stories, the boy scout/girl scout and ballerina stories. We *need* wunderkinds and we *need* TV stars!

But don't we also need to balance all the good stuff with the other reality, which is that not all of our kids are going to achieve what we hope for them no matter how hard we try to make those hopes and dreams come true? And no matter what our children achieve, there are always going to be other children who outshine them?

The mother and father who were at the clinic that day with their very slow, low-functioning son with Down syndrome had looked at Ben and Mara with more than interest. Rae and I both read in their eyes a wistfulness, a yearning: the unspoken words. . ."If only he could be as they are. . . ."

It is humbling to know that someone looks at your child and has such a wish.

What do we say to these parents? They are certainly part of us, aren't they? Don't we belong together, all of us geared to the same spectrum, no matter where upon that spectrum our kids end up?

# Time to Go?

. . . . . . . . . . . . . . . . . . . . . . .

Deep down inside where I try not to think about things, an awareness is growing that it is time for Ben to be in a group home. This is not a new thought, but one Allen and I have discussed off and on through the years when we didn't have to face it as something *real* and possibly *imminent*. But lately this awareness keeps rising to the surface whether I like it or not; I don't like it, if truth be told.

No one thing has triggered these thoughts. It's more as if a cumulation of incidents and circumstances is presenting us with a picture we cannot avoid looking at, at least not forever.

This picture has really seemed to come together during the last year or two. Last summer, for example, Allen and I rented the same apartment at the beach that we have gone to for years. Ann and Doug and his wife, Natalie, were able to join us part time. Our week was great; it usually is. (Forget the year we rented a cottage and it rained night and day without letup except for three hours in the middle of a Wednesday.) As always, we did all the fun summertime activities most people do at the beach. But we found that Ben was often reluctant to join us. He loves the ocean, and has a great time riding the waves and running along the water's edge with the gulls, or just sitting on the sand observing. Why, then, did he so often choose to remain in the apartment watching TV rather than go down to the beach with us? At home he frequently won't come when we go somewhere. But the beach? A place he looks forward to visiting for months ahead of time?

A few weeks before our family trip, Ben had spent a weekend at the beach with his Confidence Bound group. From all reports, he had participated eagerly in everything his friends and counselors did.

So what's going on here?

I think it is pretty obvious that Ben is expressing his need for independence. There are various manifestations of this need, clues which are hard to ignore, especially as we are coming to understand them.

When Ben refuses to join us and chooses instead to stay home, what does he do? Does he do something vitally necessary? Thought provoking? Challenging? Not on your life! He stays in his room alone playing records and tapes. Mostly he plays the Beatles, and although he has listened to all of his recordings countless times, he becomes indignant if we enter his room or interrupt him while he is doing this. "Privacy!" It is *his* realm and *his* music and I guess he views us as intruders.

When he is not in his room listening to music, Ben is downstairs in the rec room watching TV. His taste in TV viewing is not something I care to brag about. When Ben is not watching wrestling—the greater-than-life struggles of Hulk Hogan and cohorts—he is watching cartoons, unfortunately not the kind that are age appropriate or up to his intelligence level. If he were watching Bugs Bunny or Sylvester and Tweety Bird I'd probably be watching with him, but he watches those awful ones produced on the cheap which seem to feature a lot of robots and characters with annoying voices. If someone were to say to me, "Oh my, you shouldn't let him do that," I'd say, "Fine, you come and make this strong, determined young adult turn off the TV and engage in meaningful conversation or something else *you* think he should be doing! I'll sit back and watch."

In addition to listening to tapes and watching TV, Ben likes to sit outside our house, and, using his considerable imagination, play with his sticks and branches. These he collects in the woods on his way home from work and piles near our front porch. A stranger observing Ben with his sticks would be mystified and would almost surely conclude that he is off the wall, a real weirdo. But what Ben has done with his sticks is to invest them with personalities based on the wrestlers and the cartoon warriors from TV. With them, he conducts great battles and strategies and morality plays in which the good guy always wins! As odd as his behavior appears, it actually proves that Ben is observant, creative, and intelligent. We have mixed feelings about this particular behavior; we do not consider it exactly appropriate, but we do understand it.

Another major manifestation of Ben's desire for independence is his attitude toward food! Ben uses food in a variety of ways to exert some control over his life, as do several of his friends. Like most good Americans, Ben is enamored of french fries, hamburgers, ice cream, and soft drinks. Every chance he gets, Ben partakes of foods he knows we discourage him from eating. When given the opportunity, he eats these foods even if he's not hungry. In fact, he outright tells us he "wants to be fat!" There is absolutely no way to reason with him on this subject. In any discussion of nutrition, sensible eating, muscle tone, excess pounds—name your terminology—I would pit him against a weight-reduction "expert" any day. I can just visualize one of those weight-loss commercials with Ben in the background, fist raised in defiance and shouting, "I want to be fat!"

Ben's job adds to his eating problems. First, because he works only part time, he's home a lot. This means he has access to the refrigerator; this also means he can make himself a sandwich or snack whenever he wants, unless I spend my whole time on guard in the kitchen—something I refuse to do. Second, at work he has access to the soft-drink machine—the perfect perk—and on his breaks he has the same freedom as others to use that machine if he wishes, and oh he wishes! It is certainly not up to supervisors or fellow employees to "babysit" him. Unless he is self-motivated to control his own food habits, he is going to indulge himself. Allen and I can attempt to reason with him until we turn blue in the face without making the slightest impression on him, except to strengthen his resolve to be fat!

Now, if all this paints Ben as a gluttonous loner verging on the anti-social, it is a vastly distorted picture. When Ben is with his friends or siblings, participating in Special Olympics, and especially when he is involved with his Confidence Bound group, he is definitely "with it"—mature, cooperative, and very charming. He enjoys interacting with his fellow members and considers the counselors to be his good buddies, the best—which they are. He rises to every occasion and is more than socially adept. Ben is truly happy when he is with his friends and they are doing things together: basketball, dinner theater, swimming, a Christmas Ball.

We are very aware of these differences between Ben's behavior at home and away from home, and this awareness is telling us something.

It's not as if Allen and I have never had a child "leave the nest" before. One by one, our three older children went out on their own. (Well, almost on their own—they still come home a lot for dinner and car repairs, even the married ones.) We are not novices in saying goodbye. Why, then, is it so hard to face the thought of letting Ben go? I can scarcely bear to think of it: not to see him every day, not to hear his Beatles music, or his daily request for a tuna-fish sandwich, or his funny phone calls—I'd even miss doing his laundry. Do other parents of kids with Down syndrome feel this way? Especially mothers? Allen is not split in two the way I am. He believes it is time for Ben to go, and is ready to do something about it, although he admits it will be tough.

What about Ben himself? Ben knows what a group home is. He and his friends have visited a couple of group homes and even attended parties there. But when asked whether he would like to move into a group home, he says no, that *someday* he wants to live in an apartment. His attitude, of course, reinforces my own reluctance.

All the rational reasons that he should go are there and I can't disagree with any of them. Years ago, in fact, we put Ben's name on several waiting lists for group homes in our area. There is no reason to think, though, that they're going to have a place for him any time soon; the waiting lists are long and emergency situations are considered first. Even if we were to set things in action this very day, there would probably be a long wait. But taking that step to start the action is what I can't bring myself to do, not yet.

A few years ago, our daughter Ann was a counselor in a group home for women with mental retardation run by our local ARC. As a staff member, Ann saw to it that the residents were leading busy, happy lives. She always felt that it was a true home, not just a place. Ann is a very strong supporter of the group-home concept, and her assurances are comforting.

Still, as if to bolster what Ann tells us, I go over and over all the reasons why Ben should be in a group home. It would be best for him,

I'm fully attuned to that, probably more so than anyone. He would be with people near his own age. He would be challenged every day—far more so than he is now in spite of, or maybe because of, all that we do for him. He would be involved in more activities— night school, dinner outings, movies, shopping. A lot goes on in a group home, according to Ann. He would also be required to become more responsible for himself than he needs to be while living at home with Mom and Dad. There is no doubt he would lead a more fulfilled life partaking of the independence he so longs for.

Other young people leave home. Why shouldn't Ben?

It would be good for Allen and me too—wouldn't it? That's what the "experts" say. We would be "free!". . . . But I don't want to be "free." I have never wanted to be "free" of Ben, not really, not for any length of time. There are moments, of course, but his two weeks away at camp are about all I've ever been able to manage.

Thinking about Ben leaving home has raised a lot of questions for me, and the more raised, the more I seem to come up with. For all the talk about the value of group homes and independent living, are parents truly happy to have their children move out on their own? They may accept the change, but are they *happy*? It is so good to be *needed*—is that why it is so hard to let go?

I do not wish to be ludicrous on this subject, so bear with me. We have a cat—or more precisely, *I* have a cat—a mean, ornery animal whose name is Rotten Red, which should tell you something. Red has done some awful things, including giving me a bite on the leg that took thirteen stitches to close up. Nobody can understand why I am so attached to this cat, and they think I am crazy for keeping him. Nobody likes him; they wish him the worst. But I don't. I have saved him time and again from all kinds of disasters. If it weren't for me, he would long since have been done in and become part of a soil-replenishment spot in the backyard. The fool cat *needs* me in order to survive and *that* is the only explanation I can give for loving him, and I do love him!

I guess the desire to be needed does not always go hand in hand with common sense, or decisions we know to be right. Parents spend a great part of their lives nurturing, and to do a good job, are expected to prepare their children to reach adulthood, to "grow up," by letting them go. We are expected to do the same for our children with Down syndrome. That's how it's *supposed* to be, and it does sound fine in theory. But isn't it doubly hard to let our kids with Down syndrome go because we know that they will never be fully adult in a realistic, practical sense? Ah, but it is best, we are told, to let them go and rely on others to be as aware, as concerned, as we are. Isn't that a lot to ask of loving parents who've spent a lifetime in caring? It reminds me of the game where you are required to deliberately fall over backwards and *trust* someone *else* to catch you. It's a game I never chose to play.

When the time comes for Ben to move to a group home, chances are he will adjust very well and be truly happy. This seems to be how it usually works out. Even so, I wonder: are parents in our situation left with a deep-down gnawing feeling of missing something—or someone who *needs* them—a feeling that never quite goes away? I suspect that this is so, or will be for me.

To see Ben living a life independent of us, adjusted and busy and functioning to his full capabilities would be a joy unsurpassed. I know this to be true. Yet, oh yet, I wish we could go back to the time when years stretched ahead and we didn't have to consider what to do with another empty bedroom.

# The Saddest Words

··································· · ··················

Call me a sentimentalist, but that treacly old ballad, "Maud Muller," by John Greenleaf Whittier, still gets to me. Perhaps you remember it from high school English class—the one about the simple village maid whose life is doomed by a wrong choice. Mind you, it's not the whole poem that affects me; it's just those two lines toward the end. "For all sad words of tongue or pen, the saddest are these: It might have been!" The thing is, you see, those words are true. Let me explain.

Like most active members of parent groups, through the years I've taken a lot of phone calls from parents, grandparents, interested friends, social workers, doctors, and nurses—all kinds of people seeking information about Down syndrome, our parent group, or community resources. Most calls are pretty straightforward. Calls from new parents who are still deeply wounded must be handled very carefully, of course, but these calls are not out of the ordinary. Sometimes, though, you get a "different" kind of call, a call that leaves you disturbed and frustrated, and that haunts you forever.

One day my phone rang and when I answered it, a man's voice asked if this were the Down syndrome parent group. I said it was and identified myself. The man, who was calling long distance from another part of the state, wasted no time with preliminaries. He asked me one question: how would he go about getting a brand-new baby into Rosewood, the state institution for the mentally retarded? I remember so well the sinking feeling that came over me because his voice was so controlled, so dispassionate. I asked him about the baby—whose baby it was and why it should be sent to Rosewood. The baby was his son, only he didn't say that. What he said was, "My wife gave birth to a Mongoloid boy and I'm looking for a place that will take such a baby."

I talked to him as I had talked to so many parents before. I emphasized that he and his wife should give themselves time, that they shouldn't make any hasty decisions, that they were still in shock and might have a very different perspective in just a few weeks. He listened politely to all I had to say and when I asked him if he had any questions, the first words out of his mouth were again, "How can I get this baby into Rosewood?"

How could he even think of sending his baby to Rosewood?! I wanted to scream at him, anything to get through to him, but I kept my cool, although I was shaking.

Rosewood! Pretty name, isn't it? And it conjures up such a pretty picture—wooded glades, blooming flowers, the bucolic bliss of a gentle haven. Once Allen and I had to take Ben there for a psychological exam in connection with the research program Ben was part of.

The grounds were large and spacious enough and there were trees and some flowers, but the buildings were old and stark. We saw a playground with a dilapidated slide and broken swings; maybe it didn't matter, no one was using them. We had to climb three or four flights to the psychologist's office, the stairwell dingy with peeling paint and reeking of an awful smell. I remember seeing a young man with mental retardation wandering aimlessly on the stairs, up and down, again and again. He was there when we arrived and he was there when we left. When the appointment was over and we got back in the car, Allen and I sat there and looked at each other, both of us thinking the same thought. Never, never would we allow Ben to end up in such a place! No matter what we had to do—sell our very souls if need be—we would make sure that he did not spend his life imprisoned by neglect, aimlessly wandering on stairs that led to nowhere. I do not exaggerate when I say that being there that day and seeing firsthand what it was like scared the wits out of us.

Those who ran Rosewood did the best they could, I'm sure. But it was a *state institution*, and was exactly what the term so often implies—under-funded, under-staffed, a decaying relic from the past when people with mental retardation were warehoused and mostly forgotten. Rosewood has since been scaled down and made into one of five developmental disability centers. Many of its former residents have been moved to smaller facilities, and some lucky few have even made it into group homes.

But at the time of this particular phone call, Rosewood was still open, with one exception. No new babies were being accepted (something to be grateful for). When I told the father this he didn't respond, so I asked him about his wife, how she felt about the baby and the decision not to keep him. It was then that he told me that his wife wasn't up to making any decisions, that he and *his mother*—the baby's grandmother, only he didn't refer to her that way—were making all decisions. The picture became clearer to me now, but still I had to try. Tactfully (I think) I suggested that because Rosewood wouldn't take the baby, he might want to let some time pass and wait until he and his wife could talk things over. Again he seemed to listen, but this time his question was whether I knew of any *other* place or person who would take a new baby. At that time I did not, and this was the *only* information he was interested in. (There is now an adoption service run by a woman in White Plains, New York, with a waiting list of over a hundred families who *want* to adopt babies with Down syndrome.) He gave me his phone number in case I came up with something, and I told him to please not rush into anything, and that he or his wife could call me any time of the day or night if they needed to talk—I would be glad to help them in any way I could. He thanked me politely and hung up.

That call bothered me so. For days I thought about it, wondering particularly about the wife. What did she know about her baby? What had she been told, or not been told? Had she recovered enough to make a stand for her son, and did she even want to?

About four weeks passed. I couldn't stop thinking of them. Was it possible a change of heart had occurred and they'd decided to keep the baby? It got to the point where I could endure it no longer, so I called.

The father answered almost immediately. I identified myself and asked him how things were going. Fine. Everything had been taken care of. He didn't elaborate and I didn't want to press him. Was it possible I could speak to his wife? No, she wasn't up to it and it wouldn't be necessary anyway. My earlier suspicions were certainly confirmed; this guy did not want his wife to have one word of conversation with me! How was the baby doing? Fine, he was sure—well, he *supposed*.

Then he told me. He and his mother had found a private, out-of-state facility and had sent the baby there, and his parents—the baby's grandparents—were going to pay for it. He thanked me for calling but they didn't have a problem anymore and wouldn't be needing my help. End of conversation.

That was about a dozen or more years ago and though I never saw those people face to face, I can't forget them. I especially can't forget the grandparents, no doubt in part because since that time Allen and I have become grandparents ourselves.

Several years after the disturbing phone call, we attended a really great party, one of those parties with lots of interesting people crossing all generations. There were little kids scampering around, their parents, young singles, older folks, and some sort of in-between like us. It was a lively scene with music, wine, good food, and engaging conversation. For a time that evening, I talked with one of the young mothers while her bright-eyed baby daughter sat in an infant seat between us cooing and showing her dimples. That baby obviously loved being at the party, as did her precocious four-year-old sister, who was playing combination tag and hide-and-seek with the hostess's granddaughter. They were the cutest kids, all of them, healthy and bright and full of life!

The next day I called the hostess to thank her and tell her what a good time we'd had. I mentioned what a kick we'd gotten out of her little granddaughter and the other two, the baby and her sister.

"Yes, they're quite a pair. It's hard to believe that their grandparents have never wanted to see them."

I wasn't sure I'd heard her right. "Not want to see them? Why not?"

"Because they didn't approve of their daughter's interracial marriage and they put her and her children out of their lives."

From time to time, I find myself thinking about these two sets of grandparents who turned away from their grandchildren. No doubt they felt they had strong and compelling reasons for acting as they did. Fear or shame at seeing their own child raising a child with retardation? Standing up for what they perceived as some kind of racial principle? Reasons, perhaps, we can't begin to understand.

Did they anguish over their decision? Did they think deeply about it? Did they act in haste and bitterness just to have done with it?

I do not know these people. But I do know something about them. I know that they have let something infinitely precious slip from their lives. In today's world, where violence, cruelty, and indifference hold powerful sway, it seems to me such folly to turn our backs on those who ask nothing but to love and be loved in return, to unreservedly share their childhood: sticky kisses, first steps, a *real* train ride, visits to the pumpkin patch and the petting zoo, "fry-fries" at McDonald's, bedtime stories, a warm little body curled asleep on a lap. These grandparents— who haven't let themselves be grandparents—may never realize what they have lost. But I wonder. I wonder if sometimes they aren't aware of an empty place, a yearning, a mourning for something they can't quite pinpoint? Or can they?

The other day I was watching Ben, who has Down syndrome, and grandson, Tyler, who is biracial, roughhousing on the much-worn beanbag chair. They didn't see me, so I observed unnoticed. As usual, big old Ben was getting the worst of it from small, agile Tyler. Suddenly Tyler stopped his pummeling long enough to shout, "Ben, I love you!" "I know," Ben sighed, and raised his hands in self-defense as Tyler resumed action.

I stood chuckling to myself as I looked at them (ready to rescue Ben if need be): those two with such simpatico, whose futures will take very different paths. Already things are changing as Tyler grows and matures. Not yet three, Tyler even now is doing things that Ben is incapable of doing. But two things will never change: the common bond they share in being part of the family which so loves and needs them, and the awareness of how diminished we would be if their two dear faces were missing from our family circle.

For those who turned away, I do believe it is true that the saddest words are these: "It might have been!"

# Down Syndrome

What *is* Down syndrome and how do you "get it"?

Down syndrome is the most common clinical cause of mental retardation *and* the most common chromosomal abnormality in human beings. About six thousand babies with Down syndrome are born each year in the United States, and many thousands more throughout the world. It might be said that Down syndrome is the great equalizer. These children are born to families of all races and all economic levels. Recent research indicates that more males than females are born with Down syndrome.

Scientists do not yet know what causes the chromosomal abnormality that leads to Down syndrome. But they do know what that chromosomal abnormality *is.* In each of the millions of cells in their bodies, individuals with Down syndrome have an extra chromosome. Instead of the normal forty-six chromosomes, they have forty-seven. (Chromosomes are the microscopic, rod-shaped bodies that carry the genes, those all-important blueprints of life. Human traits such as height, body shape, eye color, and artistic tendencies are programmed in our genes.)

Down syndrome is also known as *Trisomy 21* because that fateful extra chromosome is usually located on Chromosome Pair 21. But there are two other types of Down syndrome. About 5 percent of people with Down syndrome have *Translocation Trisomy 21,* in which a part of the number 21 chromosome breaks off during cell division and attaches to another chromosome. Then there is *Mosaicism,* which affects only 1 or 2 percent of those with Down syndrome. In Mosaicism, not all cells have the extra chromosome, and that individual may have fewer charac-teristics of Down syndrome.

Although people with Down syndrome have an extra number of chromosomes, all of their other chromosomes are normal. *And* the material in the extra chromosome is also normal. Here is a prime example of what is meant by having "too much of a good thing." That additional chromosomal material results in a genetic imbalance that adversely affects both physical and mental development.

Certain features are characteristic of Down syndrome, which is why people with Down syndrome may seem to resemble one another. For example, in some people with Down syndrome, the bridge of the nose is flatter and the nose is smaller, often giving the face a flat appearance. Nasal passages may also be smaller. The mouth too may be small, and the roof of the mouth shallow. Poor muscle tone is also frequently a problem, and can result in a protruding tongue. Ears may be small and even set lower on the head. One of the readily identifiable features is the slanting eyes, which in the past gave rise to the term *Mongolism.* There are other differences (doctors have recorded over one hundred) which may not be so obvious at first glance, but which experts can usually spot right away. For example, more than 40 percent of babies with Down syndrome are born with heart defects, and many have hearing or visual impairments. Most significantly, Down syndrome causes mental retardation.

Not all individuals with Down syndrome have all these characteristics. The degree of mental retardation also varies a great deal, but is usually in the mild to moderate range. Most people with Down syndrome are quite capable of learning. And what they learn, they remember.

Women over the age of thirty-five face an increased risk of giving birth to a baby with Down syndrome, and the risk goes up with age. At age forty, the risk is 1 in 110 births; at age 45, it is 1 in 35. Many babies with Down syndrome are also born to very young mothers.

But, it can happen to anyone.

For more information about Down syndrome, contact the following organizations:

Association for Retarded Citizens
P.O. Box 1047
Arlington, TX 76004

National Down Syndrome Congress
1800 Dempster Street
Park Ridge, IL 60068–1146

National Down Syndrome Society
141 Fifth Avenue
New York, NY 10010

# About the Author

. . . . . . . . . . . . . . . . . . . . . . . . . . . . . . . . . . . .

Marilyn Trainer is a contributing author of *Babies with Down Syndrome*. Her previous essays and articles have been widely published, appearing in *The Washington Post*, *The Washington Star*, *The Humanist*, and *Your New Baby* among other publications. The mother of four, Trainer and her husband, Allen, make their home in Silver Spring, MD. This is her first book.